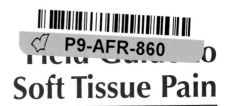

Field Guide to Soft Tissue Pain

Diagnosis and Management

Field Guide to Soft Tissue Pain

Diagnosis and Management

Robert W. Simms, M.D.
Associate Professor of Medicine
Clinical Director of Rheumatology
Boston University School of Medicine
Boston, Massachusetts

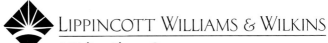

LIPPINCOTT WILLIAMS & WILKINS
A **Wolters Kluwer** Company
Philadelphia · Baltimore · New York · London
Buenos Aires · Hong Kong · Sydney · Tokyo

Acquisitions Editor: Richard Winters
Developmental Editor: Pamela Sutton
Production Editor: Aureliano Vázquez, Jr.
Manufacturing Manager: Benjamin Rivera
Cover Designer: Jeane E. Norton
Compositor: Maryland Composition Company
Printer: R. R. Donnelley, Crawfordsville

Library of Congress Cataloging-in-Publication Data

Simms, Robert W.
    Field guide to soft tissue pain: diagnosis and management/Robert W. Simms.
        p. ; cm.
    Includes bibliographical references and index.
    ISBN 0-7817-1647-0 (alk. paper)
        1. Soft tissue injuries. 2. Pain. 3. Nonarticular rheumatism. 4. Fibromyalgia.
    5. Myalgia. I. Title
        [DNLM: 1. Joint Disease—diagnosis. 2. Joint Diseases—therapy.
    3. Pain—diagnosis. 4. Pain—therapy. WE 304 S592f2000]
    RC925.5 .S46 2000
    616.7—dc21
                                                                                    00-055877

Care has been taken to confirm the accuracy of the information presented and to describe generally accepted practices. However, the author and publisher are not responsible for errors or omissions or for any consequences from application of the information in this book and make no warranty, expressed or implied, with respect to the currency, completeness, or accuracy of the contents of the publication. Application of this information in a particular situation remains the professional responsibility of the practitioner.

The author and publisher have exerted every effort to ensure that drug selection and dosage set forth in this text are in accordance with current recommendations and practice at the time of publication. However, in view of ongoing research, changes in government regulations, and the constant flow of information relating to drug therapy and drug reactions, the reader is urged to check the package insert for each drug for any change in indications and dosage and for added warnings and precautions. This is particularly important when the recommended agent is a new or infrequently employed drug.

Some drugs and medical devices presented in this publication have Food and Drug Administration (FDA) clearance for limited use in restricted research settings. It is the responsibility of the health care provider to ascertain the FDA status of each drug or device planned for use in their clinical practice.

10 9 8 7 6 5 4 3 2 1

Dedicated to my wife Linda, and my sons,
Christopher and Jeremy

Contents

Preface

Field Guide to Soft Tissue Pain: Diagnosis and Management was written with the principal aim of providing a guide to primary care physicians and caregivers in the practical diagnosis and treatment of patients with soft tissue pain. Soft tissue pain encompasses a broad array of disorders involving tendons, bursae, ligaments, and muscle. Since related conditions involving intervertebral discs, cartilage, and nerves commonly overlap with true soft tissue disorders, these are also included here. Each chapter details relevant functional anatomy and covers regional anatomic organization from the neck to the feet. An additional chapter is devoted to fibromyalgia, perhaps best considered a generalized form of soft tissue rheumatism. Finally, the last chapter covers the practical application of soft tissue injections, an integral treatment modality in management.

I owe special thanks to my wife, Linda, and my two boys, Jeremy and Christopher, who have permitted me the time to write this book. Without their patience and support its completion would have been impossible. I also owe a debt of gratitude to my colleagues in the Rheumatology Section of Boston University School of Medicine, especially Drs. Burt Sack, Peter Merkel, and Joseph Korn, who provided helpful guidance.

Robert W. Simms, M.D.

Field Guide to Soft Tissue Pain

Diagnosis and Management

1

⟳ Neck Pain

Neck pain is second only to low back pain in symptom prevalence in the general population. Neck pain may be categorized in a similar fashion as low back pain because it may result from mechanical or muscular causes, including myofascial pain, or less frequently from medical illnesses, such as degenerative disc disorders, herniation of the disc, and various forms of arthritis. The evaluation of the patient with neck pain should focus on delineating the potential process and directing a course of management.

FUNCTIONAL ANATOMY

The cervical spine is comprised of vertebral bodies vertically configured in much the same way as the lumbar spine, with several important modifications. The transverse processes of C-1 through C-6 are punctured by the foramen transversarium, through which travels each vertebral artery. The first and second cervical vertebrae represent unique vertebral levels that facilitate articulation with the skull (Fig. 1.1). Like the lumbar vertebrae, the cervical vertebrae contain zygapophyseal joints, formed from articular processes of contiguous vertebrae, and comprised of a surface of articular cartilage and a fibrous capsule (Fig. 1.2). The atlas, C-1, has no vertebral body. It resembles a bony ring with thickened lateral margins that contain articular facets, articulating inferiorly with the axis, C-2, and superiorly with the condyles of the occiput. The atlas forms a platform on which the skull rests, and its unique configuration permits axial rotation of the skull, which moves with the atlas as a single unit. Normal movement of the cervical spine includes 70 to 90 degrees of lateral rotation, 70 to 90 degrees of extension, 90 degrees of flexion, and a minimum of 45 degrees of lateral bending. The odontoid process of the axis forms a pseudovertebral body around which the atlas rotates. The odontoid process articulates with the atlas via synovial joints, which allow a large range of axial rotation. A series of ligaments attach the atlas to the occiput extending from both the anterior and posterior longitudinal ligaments. The zygapophyseal joints of the cervical spine are similar to those of the lumbar spine. They are formed by the inferior articular process of one vertebra and the ipsilateral superior articular process of the next.

The **neural anatomy** is particularly important in the evaluation of cervical spine disorders (Table 1.1). The sensory dermatomes correspond to the following cervical chord levels: C-5 the lateral portion of the deltoid (Fig. 1.3), C-6 the thumb and radial forearm (Fig. 1.4), C-7 the middle finger, and C-8 the hypothenar area. Motor functions correspond to the following levels: C-5 deltoid, C-6 biceps, C-7 triceps, C-8 finger flexors, and T-1 interossei. For the deep tendon re-

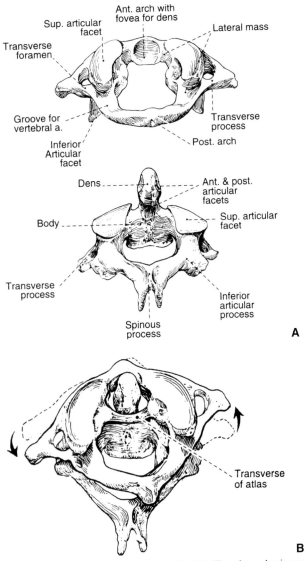

Figure 1.1 A: The atlas and axis seen from behind. **B:** The atlas and axis seen together.

Neck Pain

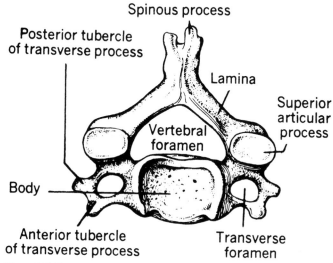

Figure 1.2 View of the fourth cervical vertebra, superior aspect.

Table 1.1   Neurology of the Upper Extremity

Disc	Root	Reflex	Muscles	Sensation
C4-5	C5	Biceps reflex	Deltoid Biceps	Lateral arm
C5-6	C6	Brachioradialis reflex (biceps reflex)	Wrist extension Biceps	Lateral forearm
C6-7	C7	Triceps reflex	Wrist flexors Finger extension Triceps	Middle finger
C7-1	C8	—	Finger flexion Hand intrinsics	Medial forearm
T1-2	T1	—	Hand intrinsics	Medial arm

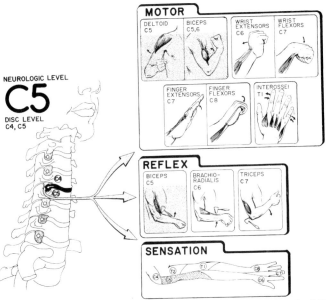

Figure 1.3 A herniated disc between vertebrae C-4 and C-5 involves the C-5 nerve root.

flexes, the biceps corresponds to C-5, the brachioradialis to C-6, and the triceps to C-7.

DIFFERENTIAL DIAGNOSIS

Neck pain has myriad potential causes that reflect the numerous anatomic structures of the cervical spine and the close approximation of the upper extremities and the thorax. Neck pain of spinal origin also may originate from many pathologic conditions, including cervical nerve root compression from herniated discs or degenerative spondylosis, cervical radiculitis, brachial plexitis, peripheral nerve entrapment syndromes, and peripheral neuropathies. It should be noted that pain originating from cervical structures can cause pain that is referred segmentally to the upper extremities and often is confused with radiculopathy. This so-called "sclerotomal" pattern of referred pain is poorly understood and frequently defies anatomic delineation. In fact, ill-defined cervical pain syndromes constitute the most common cause of neck pain and, in that sense, are similar to the lumbar spine. Similar to the lumbar spine, "mechanical" factors are responsible for the bulk of

Neck Pain

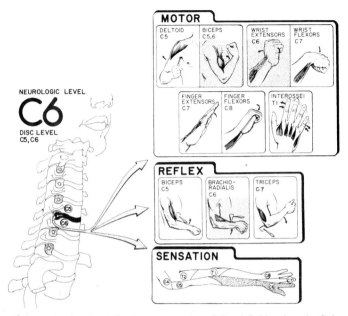

Figure 1.4 A herniated disc between vertebrae C-5 and C-6 involves the C-6 nerve root. This is the most common level of disc herniation in the cervical spine.

neck pain disorders, with medical conditions such as infections, inflammatory arthritis, or neuropathies constituting a minority (Table 1.2).

EVALUATION

The approach to the evaluation of the patient with neck pain is similar to the evaluation of the patient with low back pain. A detailed history should include information about the location, quality, radiation, and aggravating and alleviating factors of neck pain. The initial evaluation should focus on determining whether the symptoms are **radicular** or **nonradicular**.

> **Key Decision Point:** Neck pain should be categorized as either radicular or nonradicular. Radicular neck pain should prompt magnetic resonance imaging of the cervical spine.

Table 1.2   Differential Diagnosis of Neck Pain

Mechanical Causes of Neck Pain	Medical/Nonmechanical Neck Pain

Neck pain, nonspecific
  Cervical myofascial
    pain
  Whiplash injury
  Cervical spondylosis
	Infection
	Neoplasm
	
	Inflammatory arthritis
	Referred pain (e.g., originating
	    from the shoulder)
	Brachial neuritis
	Entrapment neuropathies of the
	    upper extremity (e.g., carpal
	    tunnel syndrome)

RADICULAR NECK PAIN

Of the causes of neck pain listed in Table 1.1, **radicular neck pain is produced most frequently by cervical spondylosis**. Radicular pain is suggested by pain radiating into the upper extremity or scapula region, often accompanied by numbness and tingling in a sensory dermatome distribution. Occasionally, radiating pain may involve the pectoral area, mimicking angina pectoris. **Spondylosis produces radiculopathy generally by one of two mechanisms: acute lateral disc herniation or lateral osteophytic outgrowth**. Although the latter condition presumably occurs over a period of time (required to produce the bony overgrowth as the result of disc degeneration), these two conditions are virtually impossible to distinguish clinically in that both may appear abruptly. Cervical spondylosis results from progressive deterioration of the cervical intervertebral disc, in which the inner nucleus pulposus loses its avidity for water and compresses as the result of the weight of the head. With loss of disc height, there is progressive wear on the facet and uncovertebral joints, leading to cartilage loss and osteophyte formation. In most cases, cervical spondylosis is asymptomatic, or perhaps only limitation of cervical motion is the only detectable sign. Alternately, nonradicular cervical spondylosis may produce deep pain localized to the lower posterior cervical spine.

Infrequently, radicular cervical spondylosis may present with only muscle weakness and atrophy in the distribution of the involved nerve root. The C-6 and C-7 nerve roots are the most commonly involved with cervical spondylosis; less frequently involved is C-5. Physical examination of patients with radicular cervical spondylosis may be characterized by both nonspecific and specific signs. Nonspecific signs of cervical radiculopathy include limitation of passive motion of the cer-

Neck Pain

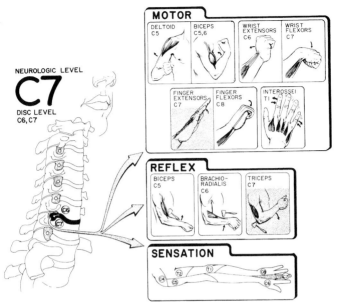

Figure 1.5 A herniated disc between vertebrae C-6 and C-7 involves the C-7 nerve root.

vical spine, tenderness, and increased pain with deviation of the neck to the side of the nerve root compression due to narrowing of the neural foramina. Specific localizing signs of C6-7 space radiculopathy (approximately 60% of cervical radiculopathies) include loss of the triceps tendon reflex, triceps weakness, and atrophy (Fig. 1.5). Sensory loss may involve the index and middle fingers. Localizing signs of C5-6 space radiculopathy (30% of cases) include biceps muscle weakness, decreased biceps and brachioradialis reflexes, and sensory loss in the thumb and index finger. Involvement of the C7-T1 interspace (less than 5% of cases) produces pain and dysesthesias in an ulnar distribution with intrinsic hand muscle weakness and atrophy (Figs. 1.6 and 1.7). **Radicular neck pain warrants urgent diagnostic imaging with magnetic resonance imaging (MRI). If neural compression is confirmed, neurologic or neurosurgical evaluation is warranted**.

NONRADICULAR NECK PAIN

Most neck pain is nonradicular, and in most cases a precise pathoanatomic diagnosis is not possible. This condition is best designated as nonspecific or nonradicular neck pain. **Two subcategories**

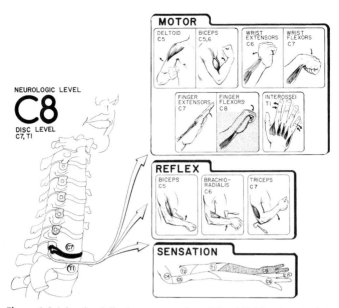

Figure 1.6 A herniated disc between vertebrae C-7 and T-1 involves the C-8 nerve root.

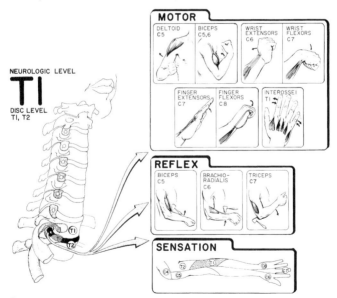

Figure 1.7 A herniated disc between vertebrae T-1 and T-2 involves the T-1 nerve root. A herniated disc in this area is unusual.

consist of **(a) whiplash injury** and **(b) myofascial pain**. The general condition, nonspecific neck pain, produces posterior or lateral neck pain that may radiate to the periscapular region or upper arm. The onset of symptoms usually is sudden, but may be more insidious on occasion, especially when associated with repetitive or occupational factors. Local muscle tenderness is the most common feature on physical examination and may occur in the suboccipital muscle, the upper trapezius, scalenes, rhomboids, and levator scapulae. The range of neck motion often is normal, although motion, especially lateral bending away from the symptomatic muscle, may produce pain.

Whiplash injury is one of the most common causes of acute neck pain. Most frequently it is caused by an acceleration-deceleration force transfer to the neck, typically during a rear-end automobile collision. Whiplash injuries may result in bony or soft tissue injuries, especially at the C5-6 level, and infrequently may produce disc herniation and radiculopathy (Table 1.3), grade III), although most patients who have chronic symptoms following a whiplash-type injury have pain that appears to originate from the zygapophyseal or facet joints.

Cervical myofascial pain is a form of nonspecific neck pain characterized by chronic neck pain without signs of radiculopathy. It is associated with localized muscle tenderness, in which palpation reproduces or accentuates the pain. Symptoms may be caused by postural

Table 1.3 Classification of Whiplash-associated Disorders

Grade	Clinical Presentation
0	No complaint about the neck
	No physical signs
I	Neck complaint of pain, stiffness, or tenderness only
	No physical signs
II	Neck complaint and musculoskeletal signs(s)[a]
III	Neck complaint and neurologic signs[b]
IV	Neck complaint and fracture or dislocation

[a] Musculoskeletal signs include decreased range of motion and point tenderness.
[b] Neurologic signs include decreased or absent deep tendon reflexes, weakness, and sensory loss.

From the Scientific Monograph of the Quebec Task Force on Whiplash-Associated Disorders. *Spine* 1995;20[8S]:1–58S.

strain or repetitive head movements. Most patients have lower posterior neck discomfort that typically is worse after rest or immobility. Paresthesias of the neck and shoulder girdle are common, although radicular signs are absent. Cervical myofascial pain is associated with other chronic musculoskeletal pain conditions such as temporomandibular joint dysfunction and fibromyalgia syndrome. In cases where symptoms are chronic and suggestive of radiculopathy even in the absence of clear signs, MRI generally is indicated to exclude cervical nerve root compression with certainty. The MRI provides more information about the soft tissue and disc anatomy than computerized tomographic scans. Plain x-rays add little to the evaluation of the patient in whom radiculopathy is considered.

MANAGEMENT

Radicular Neck Pain

Radicular neck pain generally requires specialty referral to neurology or neurosurgery. If surgery is not required immediately (usually for progressive neurologic deficits), most patients are treated with cervical support (typically a rigid support such as a Philadelphia collar), analgesics, and physical therapy. Cervical traction occasionally is recommended by the neurosurgeon and generally is best administered in a supervised setting, such as in a department of physical therapy.

Nonradicular Neck Pain

The approach to nonradicular pain is best encompassed by several modalities, including intermittent use of a soft collar for support, application of local heat for chronic symptoms, and application of ice packs for more acute pain. The judicious use of analgesics and/or nonsteroidal antiinflammatory drugs may be helpful. A topical analgesic such as capsaicin, which depletes substance P, may be useful. Local injection therapy with a steroid-anesthetic combination frequently is useful in patients with cervical myofascial pain. The most commonly used combination is 1 mL of 1% lidocaine with 10 to 20 mg of methylprednisolone, administered with a no. 25 gauge needle directly into the trigger point. Attention should be paid to proper sleep posture (the ideal is the fetal position with a cervical contour pillow for optimal neck support) and work ergonomic positioning to minimize cervical strain, such as proper keyboard and screen heights for those who use computer terminals.

2 Shoulder Pain

Soft tissue disorders of the shoulders as a group comprise the most common causes of shoulder pain in the general population and rank fifth among the regional musculoskeletal disorders as causes of disability. Of the nontraumatic soft tissue disorders, conditions that affect the rotator cuff are the most frequent, especially **rotator cuff tendinitis,** with **bicipital tendinitis,** adhesive capsulitis or **frozen shoulder,** and **suprascapular nerve entrapment** occurring in decreasing order of frequency. The clinician should bear in mind that many conditions that do not anatomically involve the shoulder produce shoulder pain. These include referred pain from conditions where the primary site of pathology is the neck, chest, or abdomen. Rotator cuff and bicipital tendinitis tend to occur most frequently during middle or later life, often following unaccustomed repetitive use of the shoulder girdle. Insurance data suggest that age older than 50 years increases the risk of injury to the rotator cuff, especially in production industry occupations. Adhesive capsulitis possesses a similar age profile and, when bilateral, is especially common in individuals with diabetes.

Soft Tissue Shoulder Disorders

- Rotator cuff tendinitis
- Bicipital tendinitis
- Frozen shoulder
- Suprascapular nerve entrapment

FUNCTIONAL ANATOMY

The shoulder joint is comprised of four basic articulations: (i) the glenohumeral joint, (ii) the acromioclavicular joint, (iii) the sternoclavicular joint, and (iv) the scapulothoracic articulation. The primary articulation of the shoulder is the glenohumeral joint (Fig. 2.1). This is a multiaxial, spheroidal, ball-and-socket type of joint, although the articulating surfaces of the joint comprise a relatively small portion of the total surface area of the humeral head. The glenohumeral joint has a large range of motion permitted in part by capsular laxity, especially in the inferior region, which allows extensive elevation and rotation. The glenoid labrum (a circumferential cartilaginous rim) enhances shoulder stability.

The musculature of the shoulder controls glenohumeral motion and can be divided into deep and superficial layers, both of which form an encircling cuff of muscle around the glenohumeral joint. The deep layer consists of the rotator cuff muscles, which stabilize the humeral head within the glenoid fossa and allow the superficial layer to produce

Shoulder Pain

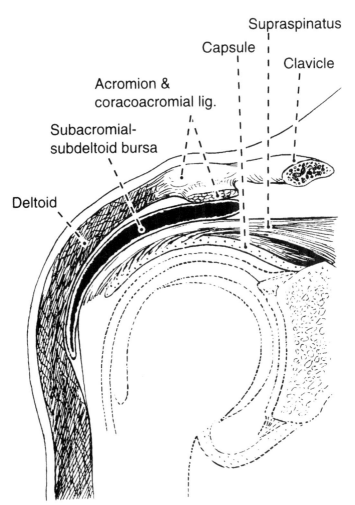

Figure 2.1 Schematic diagram of a coronal section of the shoulder region showing anatomic relations. Position of the deltoid and supraspinatus in relation to the subacromial bursa and shoulder joint capsule.

stable motion. The rotator cuff consists of the subscapularis anteriorly, the supraspinatus superiorly, and the infraspinatus and teres minor posteriorly. The biceps tendon provides additional stability interspersed between the supraspinatus and subscapularis muscles. The superficial layer consists of the deltoid, trapezius, and pectoralis muscles, which function to move the arm on the fulcrum of the distal clavicle, scapular spine, and acromion. The action of the superficial layers permits movement of the arm in three planes: anteriorly, laterally, and posteriorly. The combined action of the superficial and deep layers permits movement in these three planes as well as rotation of the arm, allowing placement of the hand above and behind the head and between the scapulae. The subacromial bursa lies between the coracocromial ligament and superior surface of the supraspinatus tendon, permitting smooth gliding of the humeral head. Inflammation of the supraspinatus tendon results in subacromial bursitis. These surfaces become adherent, producing the so-called "impingement syndrome," in which pain is produced in the region of the subacromial bursa with abduction of the arm.

Acromioclavicular Joint

The **acromioclavicular joint** is a synovial lined joint between the distal end of the clavicle and the medial acromial spine. Between these two articulating surfaces is a cartilaginous disc that permits movement of this joint. During abduction and elevation of the shoulder, the acromioclavicular joint moves only a small amount, whereas the clavicle rotates approximately 30 degrees. Full compression is applied to the joint in elevation and adduction. The joint is stabilized by several ligaments: posteriorly by the posterior transverse ligament, superiorly by the deltotrapezius fascial layer, and inferiorly by the inferior ligament.

Scapulothoracic Articulation

Scapulothoracic articulation facilitates abduction, elevation, and flexion of the glenohumeral joint. It permits sliding of the scapula across the posterolateral aspect of the rib cage. Its movements are controlled by its surrounding muscles: the serratus anterior, the rhomboids, the levator scapulae, and the trapezius.

Sternoclavicular Joint

Similar to the acromioclavicular joint, the **sternoclavicular joint** contains a cartilaginous disc that facilitates movement between the clavicle and the manubrium. Its movement is hinged and multiaxial. It is stabilized by strong ligaments anteriorly and posteriorly.

ROTATOR CUFF TENDINITIS (SUBACROMIAL BURSITIS, SUPRASPINATUS TENDINITIS, IMPINGEMENT SYNDROME)

Disorders of the rotator cuff represent overall the most common cause of shoulder pain. Although tendinitis is the term commonly applied to describe the clinical scenario referable to the rotator cuff, in reality, partial tears with tendinitis or partial tears in isolation are impossible to distinguish from pure tendinitis, even at surgery or via sophisticated imaging such as magnetic resonance imaging (MRI). Complete tears of the rotator cuff, when acute, usually are produced by significant trauma and generally can be diagnosed by examination. Chronic degenerative tears that eventually become complete, however, may be clinically difficult to distinguish from chronic tendinitis. The MRI in these settings may be indispensable in distinguishing chronic tendinitis or partial tears from complete tears.

A wide variety of conditions may affect the rotator cuff and lead to impingement of the tendon complex, including structural impingement from anomalies of the coracocromial arch, osteophytes growing from the acromioclavicular joint, or calcific deposits within the supraspinatus tendon, which result, in turn, from chronic inflammation of the tendon. The combination of partial tears and inflammation is most common in overuse settings, particularly in middle-aged individuals. In this circumstance, age-related degeneration of the rotator cuff tendon is an important risk factor for chronic impingement. Acute calcific tendinitis occurs in young adults. It presents with sudden pain in the anterior lateral aspect of the shoulder and is the result of basic calcium crystal deposition within the supraspinatus or infraspinatus tendon at the site of attachment. There are no known risk factors for identification of the syndrome.

Differential Diagnosis of Rotator Cuff Tendinitis

- Cervical spondylosis
- Bicipital tendinitis
- Articular disorders of the shoulder (involving the acromioclavicular joint, sternoclavicular joint, and glenohumeral joint)

Evaluation

A history of shoulder pain, either acute, subacute, or chronic, localized to the anterolateral aspect of the shoulder, often with radiation to the lateral upper arm and increased with abduction, should lead to suspicion of rotator cuff pathology. In contrast to pain originating from cervical spondylosis, pain from rotator cuff pathology often is worse at night and is not relieved with a neck brace. Movement of the shoulder rather than the neck typically exacerbates the symptoms. The examiner should have the patient perform active flexion and abduction of the shoulder with internal and external rotation (Fig. 2.2). Simply observing the patient remove his or her shirt provides important information about functional limitation. Inspection of the shoulder girdle should include an assessment of muscle atrophy, especially of the supraspinatus

Shoulder Pain

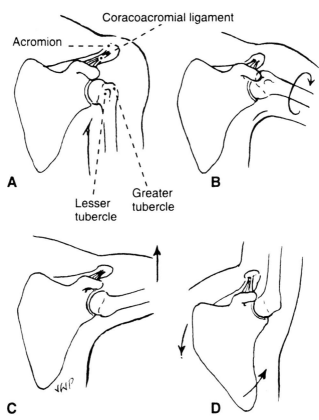

Figure 2.2 Abduction of the shoulder. Starting from the neutral position (**A**), conjunct rotation of the humerus laterally (**B, C**) places a large area of articular surface above the glenoid cavity, extending the range of glenohumoral abduction from 90 to 120 degrees. **D:** An additional 60 degrees of movement is attained by scapular rotation. (Based on McMinn RMH. *Last's anatomy,* 8th ed. London: Churchill Livingstone, 1990.)

muscle. Active movement should be formally assessed by having the patient perform four basic shoulder movements: (i) forward elevation or flexion (arm above the head); (ii) abduction (elbow flexed and abducted); (iii) external rotation and abduction (palm of hand to back of neck); and (iv) internal rotation and abduction (hand between shoulder blades). The examiner should assess passive movement of the shoulder by first stabilizing the clavicle with one hand (significant limitation of abduction can be overlooked if this is not done, because the patient can abduct the shoulder by elevating the clavicle) and then performing passive abduction and internal and external rotation. Inability to abduct actively more than 30 degrees suggests a complete tear of the rotator cuff if subsequent passive movements of the shoulder are normal. Pain, especially with progressive abduction, suggests rotator cuff pathology, because the rotator cuff, with this maneuver, is squeezed between the humeral head and the tip of the acromion and coracoacromial ligament. Another useful maneuver is to ask the patient to extend the symptomatic extremity with the thumb pointed to the floor against resistance. Pain in the shoulder suggests rotator cuff pathology. In general, rotator cuff pathology produces greater impairment of active compared to passive movement. The shoulder then should be palpated carefully to localize the region of greatest tenderness. Tenderness with rotator cuff pathology is greatest over the region of the subacromial bursa, just inferior to the most lateral portion of the acromion. Tenderness over the acromioclavicular joint and pain in this region with adduction of the arm, together with signs of rotator cuff pathology, suggest acquired impingement.

Treatment

The initial treatment of rotator cuff tendinitis should include **antiinflammatory medication, local heat** (for example, with a heating pad), and **Codman exercises** (Fig. 2.3). Local corticosteroid injection into the subacromial space is the single most effective therapy in most cases. Exercises should be resumed 48 hours after injection and should be continued for 2 weeks. A second injection can be performed at that time if there is transient or partial improvement following the first injection. A plain x-ray film of the shoulder generally is indicated at this point. A third injection after an additional 2-week period may be required. If little additional improvement occurs after a third injection, then an MRI of the shoulder is indicated to exclude anatomic impingement (for example, from an inferior spur originating from the acromioclavicular joint or a significant tear of the tendon).

Key Decision Point: Perform MRI of the shoulder if conservative treatment measures, including local injection of corticosteroid into the subacromial bursa, fail.

BICIPITAL TENDINITIS

Bicipital tendinitis results from inflammation of the sheath of the long head of the biceps along its course proximally near the insertion in the bicipital groove. The short head of the biceps tendon attaches to the coracoid process, but seldom develops tendinitis and is not important clinically. Most often, bicipital tendinitis results from impingement of

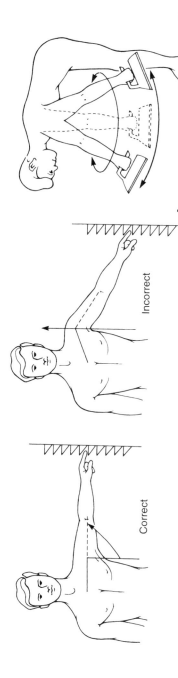

Figure 2.3 A: Correct and incorrect use of "wall-climbing" exercise. The wall-climbing exercise frequently is done improperly. The normal arm climbs with normal scapulohumeral rhythm. If there is pericapsulitis, the wall climb in abduction is done with "shrugging" of the scapula and accomplishes nothing. The wall climb should be started with the patient facing the wall and gradually turning the body until the patient is at a right angle to the wall. (Redrawn from Cailliet R. *Shoulder pain*. Philadelphia: FA Davis, 1973.) **B:** Active pendular glenohumeral exercise (so-called Codman exercises). The arm moves in a forward-and-backward sagittal plane, in forward and backward flexion. Circular motion in the clockwise and counterclockwise direction also is done in increasingly larger circles.

17

the long head by the acromion and frequently is associated with rotator cuff tendinitis or glenohumeral instability. Overuse of the affected extremity is a frequent precipitant.

> *Differential Diagnosis of Bicipital Tendinitis*
>
> • Rotator cuff tendinitis
> • Cervical spondylosis
> • Articular disorders of the shoulder

Evaluation

The clinical picture consists of anterior shoulder pain and is increased with overhead activities. Passive range of motion is normal. Bicipital pain can be reproduced by supination of the forearm against resistance with the elbow flexed to 90 degrees (Yergason's sign) (Fig. 2.4) or by flexion of the elbow against resistance. Radiographs of the shoulder are of little benefit.

Treatment

Treatment of bicipital tendinitis is similar to that of rotator cuff tendinitis. Initial therapy should include antiinflammatory medication, local heat, and Codman exercises. Local injection of corticosteroid

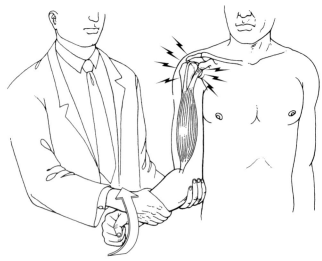

Figure 2.4 Yergason's test for bicipital tendonitis.

into the bicipital sheath is beneficial in most cases. Care should be taken not to inject directly into the tendon itself, because this can lead to rupture of the tendon. Excessive resistance to injection of corticosteroid may indicate that the needle is in the tendon and should be withdrawn before additional material is instilled. Injection into the vicinity of the tendon sheath probably is sufficient. Infrequently, more than one injection is necessary if little or partial improvement occurs with a single injection.

FROZEN SHOULDER (ADHESIVE CAPSULITIS, PERIARTHRITIS OF THE SHOULDER, PERICAPSULITIS)

Frozen shoulder, also termed adhesive capsulitis or pericapsulitis, is used to describe **restriction of shoulder movement in all three planes resulting from loss of volume of the shoulder capsule when the glenohumeral joint itself is normal.** The disorder most commonly is associated with a period of immobility of the shoulder that can result from diverse causes, including rotator cuff tendinitis, bicipital tendinitis, hemiparesis, trauma, or shoulder surgery. Loss of mobility of the shoulder joint appears to result in shrinkage of the large capsule of the glenohumeral joint, which in turn leads to progressive loss of motion. **The disorder also is associated with certain metabolic conditions, including diabetes and hypothyroidism.** In the case of diabetes, frozen shoulder may be bilateral. Initial histologic changes include increased vascularity, scattered inflammatory infiltrates, and fibroblast proliferation, followed by fibrous thickening of the capsular folds, recesses, and ligamentous structures. Adherence of the axillary pouch to the humerus results in significant loss of movement.

The onset of frozen shoulder usually is insidious and is associated with progressive limitation of movement and pain diffusely around the joint. The outcome of untreated frozen shoulder is eventual improvement in pain with residual variable limitation of movement.

Differential Diagnosis of Frozen Shoulder
- Glenohumeral arthritis
- Rotator cuff tendinitis
- Bicipital tendinitis

Evaluation

The typical finding is initial loss of external motion; however, motion also is impaired to some extent in abduction and internal rotation. Both passive and active motion are equally impaired, in contrast to other shoulder disorders of soft tissue such as rotator cuff tendinitis, in

Shoulder Pain

which limitation of movement is primarily active. Tenderness usually is diffuse around the capsule of the shoulder, and wasting of the deltoid and supraspinatus muscles can be profound. Shoulder x-ray films usually are normal or may show mild osteopenia. Diabetes and thyroid disease should always be considered, especially when frozen shoulder is bilateral.

Treatment

No single treatment modality is successful in frozen shoulder. At a minimum, most experts recommend local corticosteroid injection and physical modalities. Joint distention, nerve blocks, and manipulation under anesthesia also have been recommended. There are few controlled trials of therapy in frozen shoulder.

Local injection should include both glenohumeral and subacromial bursal injection of corticosteroid to allow the capsule to be exposed to maximal quantities of corticosteroid medication. If two sets of injections within the first 4 to 6 weeks of treatment fail to result in improvement, then oral corticosteroids for several weeks should be considered at doses such as 20 to 40 mg per day of prednisone. An exercise program consisting of active exercises, such as Codman exercises, and passive exercises, such as those administered by a physical therapist, are integral to the treatment of frozen shoulder.

> **Key Decision Point:** Consider short-term, intermediate-dose (20 to 40 mg per day of prednisone for 2 to 3 weeks) oral corticosteroids for frozen shoulder if local injection and exercise therapies fail to result in improvement within 4 to 6 weeks.

SUPRASCAPULAR NERVE ENTRAPMENT

Before the suprascapular nerve passes through the suprascapular notch, it innervates the supraspinatus muscle, the acromioclavicular (AC) joint, the glenohumeral joint, and the coracoacromial ligament. After passing through the suprascapular notch, the nerve innervates the infraspinatus muscle. Entrapment of the suprascapular nerve may occur as it passes through the notch of the scapular spine or in the spinoglenoid notch (in which case only the infraspinatus will be affected), usually from direct trauma or by ganglia. Typical symptoms are dull posterior and lateral shoulder pain.

Evaluation

The suprascapular notch is located 2 to 3 cm lateral to the midpoint of the scapula spine, and tenderness is found at this point. Weakness of shoulder abduction and external rotation typically is present, although supraspinatus or infraspinatus atrophy is a late finding. The diagnosis may be confirmed by electromyography.

Treatment

Physical therapy for 1 to 2 months is initially recommended. Local corticosteroid injection by an experienced clinician may be effective. Lack of response warrants consideration of surgical release by an orthopedic surgeon.

3   ↳ Elbow Pain

Soft tissue disorders in the elbow may be the result of **lateral epicondylitis, medial epicondylitis,** or **olecranon bursitis.** Of these, lateral epicondylitis or tennis elbow is easily the most common and may affect up to 3% of the population. It occurs primarily during middle age and is common among those who do not play tennis. Risk factors include repetitive movements of the forearm, especially repetitive wrist turning, hand gripping, tool use, or hand shaking. Tennis elbow therefore is an occupational hazard among carpenters, gardeners, dentists, and even politicians. It is, of course, a common injury among tennis players, especially beginners. Recurrent symptoms within 18 months of diagnosis are characteristic in the majority of patients.

Soft Tissue Disorders of the Elbow
- Lateral epicondylitis
- Medial epicondylitis
- Olecranon bursitis
- Ulnar entrapment neuropathy

FUNCTIONAL ANATOMY

The elbow is a compound hinged joint that permits flexion and extension as well as rotation of the forearm. **The elbow comprises three articulations: the humeroulnar joint (also known as the trochlea joint), the humeroradial joint, and the superior or proximal radioulnar joint.** The humeroulnar joint provides a uniaxial hinge between the trochlea of the humerus and the ulnar trochlear notch. The humeroradial joint is a modified uniaxial hinge joint, because it permits rotation as well as flexion and extension (Fig. 3.1). The radial head turns on the capitulum of the humerus with supination and pronation of the forearm. The three joints of the elbow share a common capsule that also includes the olecranon, coronoid, and radial fossae of the humerus, as well as the tips of the olecranon and coronoid processes. The elbow is one of the most inherently stable joints, in large part due to the depth of the trochlear notch. It also is stabilized by extensive supporting ligaments: the ulnar and radial collateral ligaments and the annular ligament. The flexors of the elbow are the biceps, which attaches to the radial tuberosity (because it attaches to the medial side of the radius, it also acts as a supinator), the brachialis, and the brachioradialis. The main extensor of the elbow is the triceps, with its attachment to the olecranon. Pronation of the forearm is accomplished by the pronator teres. The finger and wrist flexors attach to the medial epicondyle and include the flexor carpi radialis, palmaris longus, and flexor carpi ul-

Elbow Pain

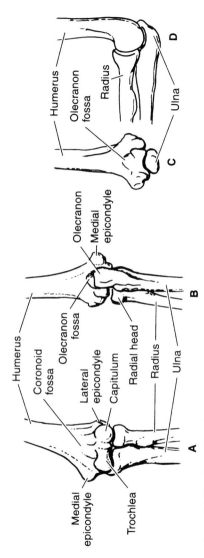

Figure 3.1 The elbow joint. **A:** Anterior view. **B:** Posterior view. **C:** Posterior view, 90 degrees flexion. **D:** Lateral view.

Elbow Pain

naris. This is the site of pain associated with medial epicondylitis. The finger and wrist extensors originate at the lateral epicondyle and include the extensor carpi radialis brevis and longus. Their origin is the usual site of pain in lateral epicondylitis. The olecranon bursa overlies the olecranon prominence, forming a superficial bursa that does not communicate with the joint. The most commonly involved neural structure of the elbow is the ulnar nerve, which passes through the medial paraolecranon groove, an exposed location for entrapment and trauma (Fig. 3.2).

LATERAL EPICONDYLITIS

The most common soft tissue disorder of the elbow is lateral epicondylitis, also known as tennis elbow. This condition typically presents as pain over the lateral aspect of the elbow and is exacerbated by wrist and finger extension. The onset of symptoms often occurs following unaccustomed activity or overuse, although precipitating factors are not always identified. A common cause is typing at a keyboard, especially if the keyboard is elevated above the level of the elbows, which tends to put excessive stress at the origin of the wrist extensors. The pathophysiology of lateral epicondylitis is not fully understood. Pathologic studies have documented tendinitis or tendon tears of the common extensor tendon attachment to the lateral epicondyle. Swelling usually is absent. Tenderness is localized just over the lateral epicondyle and increases with wrist extension against resistance. Passive movement of the elbow is normal.

Management

Treatment of lateral epicondylitis consists of rest from the precipitating activity, application of heat or ice, and nonsteroidal antiinflammatory drugs. Bands or straps worn over the proximal forearm alter the direction of muscle pull and reduce the effective length of the extensors, reducing the traction at the origin of the extensors. Local injection of corticosteroid into the anterior region of the lateral epicondyle provides relief for most patients. Following initial improvement, long-term therapy should include continued extensor stretching and strengthening exercises, such as repeated wrist extensions with light weights. Most patients improve within 1 year; rarely, persistent symptoms require surgical treatment with release of the common extensor tendon, excision of granulation tissue, or distal tenotomy to lengthen the common extensor tendon.

MEDIAL EPICONDYLITIS

Medial epicondylitis, also known as golfer's elbow, is less common and less disabling than lateral epicondylitis. It commonly occurs in

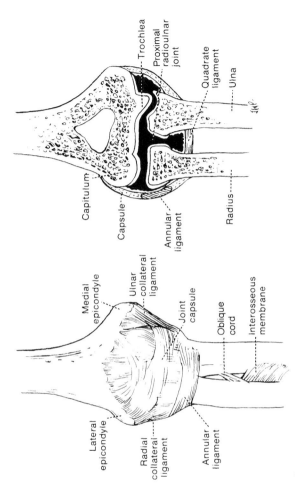

Figure 3.2 The elbow joint. **Left:** The joint capsule with its associated ligaments. **Right:** Coronal section of the joint shows the relation of the proximal radioulnar joint to the elbow. Synovial fluid is *black*.

those who engage in cumulative repetitive strain of the common flexors of the forearm, such as occurs in golfing, baseball pitching, or work-related activities. The pathology is believed to be similar to that of lateral epicondylitis. Pain onset typically is insidious and localized to the region of the medial epicondyle. Tenderness is localized just distal to the medial epicondyle, and pain increases with resistive flexion of the wrist. Swelling at the site of flexor attachment to the medial epicondyle is uncommon.

Treatment consists of rest, local ice or heat, nonsteroidal antiinflammatory drugs, or local corticosteroid injection. Wrist curls with light weights should be started after symptoms subside. Rarely, surgical release of the common forearm flexor tendon is necessary in those with chronic symptoms.

OLECRANON BURSITIS

A variety of conditions may affect the olecranon bursa. These include traumatic olecranon bursitis, septic olecranon bursitis, and nonseptic inflammatory olecranon bursitis. The latter may be associated with conditions such as rheumatoid arthritis, gout, or psoriatic arthritis.

Traumatic olecranon bursitis results from direct trauma to the olecranon, often from repeated leaning on the elbow or occasionally from a single blow. Pain and swelling localized to the olecranon result. **Aspiration of the olecranon bursa should be performed to exclude septic bursitis.** Aspiration should be performed at the sides of the bursa, because aspiration at the apex of the bursa may result in a sinus tract (See Chapter 10, Injection Techniques, and Fig. 10.3). Traumatic bursitis results in noninflammatory, typically bloody fluid. Treatment consists of application of local ice, padding the elbow to prevent reinjury, and antiinflammatory agents.

Septic olecranon bursitis results from local infiltration of bacteria from the skin. The most common organism is *Staphylococcus aureus,* with *Streptococcus* sp following in frequency. Septic olecranon bursitis presents with painful swelling of the olecranon, often with surrounding erythema. Active extension of the elbow may be painful (because the triceps muscle attaches to the olecranon), although passive movement typically is normal unless there is extensive soft tissue swelling. Occasionally, a septic olecranon bursa may rupture, producing extensive soft tissue swelling and erythema in the forearm mimicking cellulitis. In these circumstances, the olecranon bursa should be examined carefully and aspirated, because culture of the bursal fluid will facilitate microbiologic diagnosis. Treatment of septic olecranon bursitis consists of antibiotics (which may be given orally unless the patient is immunocompromised, or there is extensive cellulitis) and repeated closed aspiration.

Systemic inflammatory disorders, such as gout and rheumatoid arthritis, may involve the olecranon bursa. In the case of gout, the clinical presentation resembles that of septic olecranon bursitis. For this reason, the bursa should be aspirated and any fluid obtained sent for culture and crystal analysis. Gouty olecranon bursitis will show sodium urate crystals and polymorphonuclear leukocytes under microscopic examination. Occasionally, tophi will accumulate in the olecranon bursa. Treatment consists of local application of ice and antiinflammatory agents. Occasionally, local instillation of corticosteroids is necessary for resistant cases or if antiinflammatory agents are contraindicated.

Rheumatoid arthritis may involve the olecranon bursae most commonly with nodules that usually are minimally, if at all, symptomatic. If the nodules become troublesome, usually from direct trauma, local corticosteroid injection may be helpful.

Key Decision Points

1. Aspirate the bursa to exclude septic bursitis and gout.
2. If purulent fluid is obtained, begin antistaphylococcal antibiotics.
3. If septic bursitis is confirmed, repeated aspiration is required.

ULNAR ENTRAPMENT NEUROPATHY (CUBITAL TUNNEL SYNDROME)

Compression neuropathy of the ulnar nerve may be the result of local trauma or constriction of the nerve in the fibrous-osseus tunnel through which it passes. The tunnel is formed anteriorly by the medial epicondyle, the ulnar collateral ligament, and the flexor carpi ulnaris. The compression produces paresthesias in a C-8 distribution. Tinel's sign at the elbow is accomplished by light percussion of the ulnar nerve as it travels through the medial paraolecranon groove, which produces tingling in the ulnar distribution. The elbow flexion test also can be performed by holding the elbow in flexion for 5 minutes. Tingling in the ulnar distribution suggests ulnar entrapment.

4   ↘ Hand and Wrist Pain

The most common soft disorders of the hand and wrist include **carpal tunnel syndrome, de Quervain's tenosynovitis, trigger finger** or digital stenosing tenosynovitis, and **Dupuytren's contracture. Carpal tunnel syndrome is the most common peripheral neuropathy.** Carpal tunnel syndrome is most frequent in middle or advanced age and appears to result from a variety of possible anatomic (i.e., narrowing of the carpal tunnel) and physiologic factors (e.g., presence of diabetes or pregnancy) as well as patterns of use, including repetitive wrist flexion and extension. Carpal tunnel syndrome may be particularly disabling, and its early identification and treatment may prevent irreversible damage to the median nerve.

Soft Tissue Disorders of the Hand and Wrist

- Carpal tunnel syndrome
- de Quervain's tenosynovitis
- Trigger finger
- Ganglia
- Dupuytren's contracture

FUNCTIONAL ANATOMY

The hand is a complex and highly evolved anatomic structure that provides primary touch input to the human brain and enables humans to perform complex fine motor tasks, including grasping. **The hand comprises four functional units: the fixed carpal bones, which provide a stabilizing platform for three mobile units, the thumb, the index finger, and the unit comprising the middle, ring, and little fingers.** The wrist joint or radiocarpal joint is formed by the articulation of the radius and the carpal row of the scaphoid, lunate, and triquetrum (Fig. 4.1). It is stabilized superiorly and inferiorly by the radiocarpal ligaments (dorsal and palmar) and by collateral ligaments (radial and ulnar). The finger flexor tendons are each covered by tenosynovial sheaths that form a common flexor tendon sheath extending from the wrist, passing under the flexor retinaculum to approximately the mid-palm (Fig. 4.2). A series of annular pulleys anchor the flexor tendons and the surrounding sheaths to the palmar aponeurosis and connective tissue, and prevent bowing of the flexor tendons with finger contraction. The finger extensors possess less extensive tenosynovial sheaths that, unlike the flexor tendon sheaths, do not extend the entire length of the extensor tendons, but are centered around the wrist and are stabilized by the extensor retinaculum (Fig. 4.3). These combined sheaths include the common sheath of the ex-

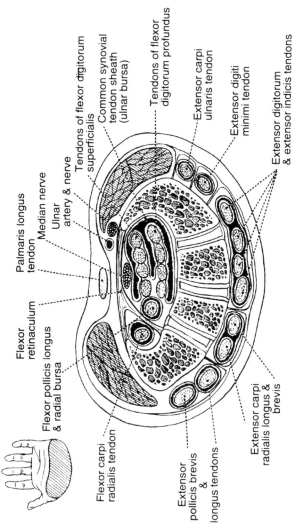

Figure 4.1 Transverse section of the wrist across the carpal canal. Synovial fluid within synovial sheaths is shown in *black*; for purposes of clarity, its quantity is exaggerated. The *inset* shows the level of the section.

Tendons of flexor digitorum superficialis

Common synovial tendon sheath (ulnar bursa)

Tendons of flexor digitorum profundus

Extensor carpi ulnaris tendon

Extensor digiti minimi tendon

Extensor digitorum & extensor indicis tendons

Palmaris longus tendon

Median nerve

Ulnar artery & nerve

Flexor retinaculum

Flexor pollicis longus & radial bursa

Flexor carpi radialis tendon

Extensor pollicis brevis & longus tendons

Extensor carpi radialis longus & brevis

Hand and Wrist Pain

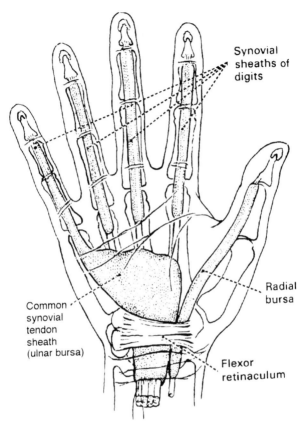

Figure 4.2 Synovial sheaths of the flexor tendons in the carpal canal and the hand. Note the proximal extent of the radial and ulnar bursae in relation to skin creases of the wrist, the upper limit of the retinaculum, and the joint line of the wrist joint. Note the relation of the digital synovial sheaths to skin creases of the palm and to the joints.

tensor pollicis brevis and abductor pollicis longus tendons and the extensor digitorum communis and extensor indicis propius.

DUPUYTREN'S CONTRACTURE

This condition is the result of **nodular thickening of the palmar fascia** producing flexion deformities of the involved digits, most commonly the fourth digit. Identified risk factors include Northern European ancestry, alcoholism, diabetes, and epilepsy. The contractures are

Hand and Wrist Pain

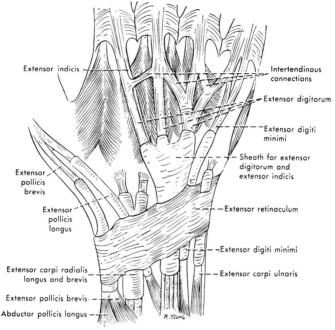

Figure 4.3 Extensor retinaculum, with the tendons and their synovial sheaths on the dorsum of the wrist.

asymptomatic and progression is quite variable. Progressive deformity and impaired hand function should prompt surgical referral for fasciectomy (Fig. 4.4).

GANGLIA

Ganglia are benign cystic lesions of the hands and wrists that appear to result most commonly from synovial outpouching or occasionally from mucinous degeneration of connective tissue followed by cavitation. Most (70%) occur on the dorsum of the wrist arising from the scapholunate and trapezium-trapezoid joints. Approximately 25% arise from between the flexor carpi radialis and brachioradialis tendons on the volar aspect of the wrist. Ganglia may present as painless, slowly growing masses, or they may be painful, rapidly appearing lesions, especially with increased hand or wrist movement (Fig. 4.5). They tend to diminish in size with rest or immobilization of the wrist. Volar wrist ganglia may result in carpal tunnel syndrome. Treatment with aspiration and corticosteroid injection is indicated for symp-

31

Hand and Wrist Pain

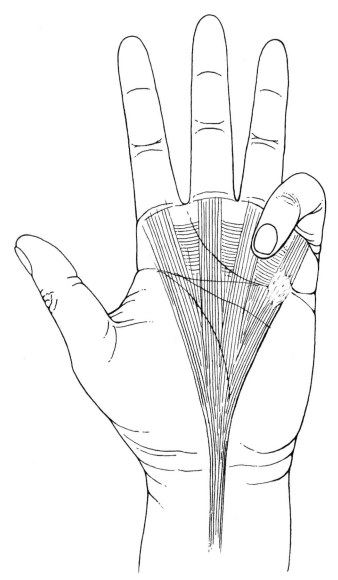

Figure 4.4 Dupuytren's contracture.

Hand and Wrist Pain

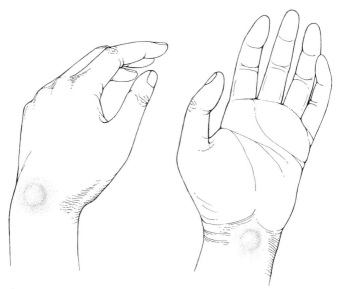

Figure 4.5 Ganglia may be found on the wrist's dorsal or volar surfaces.

tomatic ganglia. Surgical resection is indicated for large symptomatic ganglia, especially those that produce carpal tunnel syndrome.

TRIGGER FINGER (DIGITAL STENOSING TENOSYNOVITIS)

The most common repetitive soft tissue injury of the hand is so-called trigger finger. The thumb and middle finger are most commonly involved, although this condition may affect any finger. It results from **fibrosis of the flexor tendon sheath** of affected digits and is associated with repetitive fine motor tasks. Fibrosis of the circumferential tendon sheath occurs most commonly at the most proximal annular pulley (known as the A1 pulley) of the tendon sheath just distal to the transverse carpal ligament, resulting in stenosis of the sheath through which the tendon glides. Increased friction of the tendon passing through the stenotic sheath leads to pain and/or fibrotic thickening of the sheath leads to formation of a nodule that obstructs smooth gliding of the tendon and sheath through the annular pulley producing locking with flexion. Frequently, the finger must be forcibly extended by the patient. In advanced cases, the finger may be locked in flexion.

If multiple fingers are involved, diabetes, hypothyroidism, ochronosis, light-chain amyloidosis, and multicentric reticulohistiocytosis should be considered. Examination discloses a tender nodule at the palmar aspect of the metacarpophalangeal joint. Passive flexion and extension of the finger will reveal this to be the site of locking.

Treatment of trigger finger may be treated with a rest splint only, but this is relatively ineffective, with improvement in only about 20% of fingers. **Corticosteroid injection is successful with a single infiltration in approximately 60% of cases.** Surgical release is reserved for persistently locked digits or for patients who fail to improve after three injections. Care during the injection should be taken to avoid direction infiltration of the tendon, because this may result in tendon rupture (see Chapter 10 on local injection).

Trigger Finger: Key Points

1. Most commonly involves the thumb and middle finger
2. Fibrotic thickening of the flexor tendon sheath leads to locking at the annular pulleys, most commonly at the level of the metacarpophalangeal joint
3. Diabetes, hypothyroidism, and other systemic conditions should be considered when multiple digits are involved
4. Corticosteroid infiltration of the tendon sheath is the most effective therapy

---

DE QUERVAIN'S TENOSYNOVITIS

de Quervain's tenosynovitis frequently is confused with acute arthritis of the wrist. It results from inflammation of the sheath of the common extensor tendon of the thumb, combining the extensor pollicis brevis and abductor pollicis longus tendons. **de Quervain's tenosynovitis most frequently results from repetitive wrist motion in the radial or ulnar direction while pinching with the thumb.** Localized tenderness and occasionally soft tissue swelling may be found along the lateral border of the distal radius. Passive motion of the wrist is normal, but passive lateral flexion of the wrist while the patient grasps the thumb in the palm produces pain (Finkelstein's test). The differential diagnosis includes carpal tunnel syndrome, cervical radiculopathy, inflammatory arthritis of the wrist, and osteoarthritis of the carpometacarpal joint.

Treatment includes splinting of the wrist and thumb (a simple gutter plaster splint on the radial border of the distal forearm, wrist, and thumb suffices), application of local heat, and nonsteroidal antiinflammatory agents. Avoiding repetitive thumb movements is helpful. Local installation of corticosteroid into the tendon sheath is effective in most persistent cases.

> ### de Quervain's Tenosynovitis: Key Points
>
> 1. Results from inflammation of the common sheath of the extensor pollicis brevis and abductor pollicis longus tendons
> 2. Diagnosis is confirmed with a positive Finkelstein's test (pain with passive lateral flexion of the wrist while the patient grasps the thumb in the palm)

CARPAL TUNNEL SYNDROME

Carpal tunnel syndrome results from compression of the median nerve in the wrist inferior to the flexor retinaculum. It can be the result of multiple etiologies, including tendinitis of the wrist and finger flexors, synovitis of the wrist, or metabolic conditions that result in fluid accumulation in the flexor compartment (e.g., pregnancy, hypothyroidism). **The most common cause of carpal tunnel syndrome is flexor tendinitis.** This condition is **increasingly seen in users of computer keyboards,** especially when the keyboard height is higher than the elbows, a situation that ergonometrically produces excess strain on the wrist flexors. Compression of the median nerve produces numbness, tingling, or pain in the thumb, forefinger, and middle finger, although frequently dysesthesias are felt in all the digits. Patients frequently complain of nocturnal exacerbation of symptoms (frequently relieved by shaking the hand) and of dropping objects. Occasionally, carpal tunnel syndrome is mimicked by higher level impingement of the median nerve, such as cervical radiculopathy or entrapment in the proximal forearm (pronator syndrome). Reproduction of the patient's symptoms occur with percussion over the volar wrist distal to the skin crease (Tinel's sign) (Fig. 4.6), or by asking the patient to flex both wrists against each other for 1 minute (Phalen's sign) (Fig. 4.7). Reduced pinprick sensation or more commonly two-point discrimination in the median nerve distribution is found. A late sign of carpal tunnel syndrome is atrophy of the thenar eminence or weakness of thumb abduction.

Treatment of carpal tunnel syndrome includes nocturnal wrist splinting in the neutral position, antiinflammatory agents, and corticosteroid injection. In the case of flexor tendinitis, these measures combined with appropriate ergonomic adjustments (e.g., reducing the keyboard height) usually results in significant improvement in the majority of cases. Persistent symptoms despite these measures and correction of any underlying complicating condition (such as hypothyroidism) may require surgical referral for decompression.

Hand and Wrist Pain

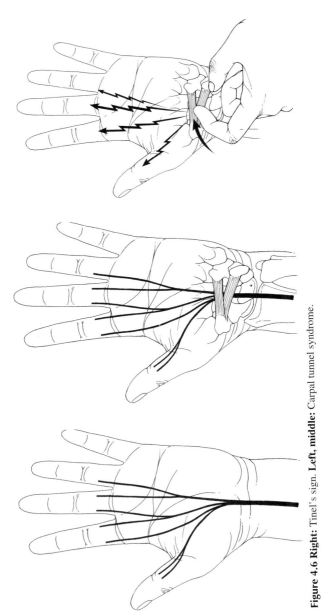

Figure 4.6 Right: Tinel's sign. **Left, middle:** Carpal tunnel syndrome.

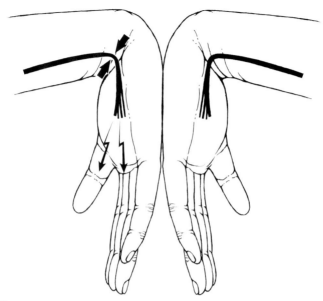

Figure 4.7 Phalen's test to reproduce symptoms of carpal tunnel syndrome.

Carpal Tunnel Syndrome: Key Points

1. Symptoms of pain and paresthesia in median nerve distribution, although they may involve all five digits
2. Nocturnal exacerbation
3. Most commonly due to flexor tendinitis ("idiopathic")
4. Positive Phalen's and Tinel's signs
5. Electromyographic and nerve conduction velocity are indicated in resistant cases, especially before surgical evaluation

5   ➲ Low Back Pain

Low back pain is among the most common symptoms to affect human beings: up to two thirds of all individuals will experience low back pain during their lifetime. Chronic low back pain accounts for nearly 13 million physician visits each year. In most cases of acute or chronic low back pain, a precise anatomic diagnosis is not possible, although most cases of low back pain can be designated as mechanical in origin. Mechanical back pain refers to that related to overuse or biomechanical injury of an anatomic structure and accounts for approximately 90% of all causes of back pain. The remaining 10% of back pain is the result of medical illnesses, such as osteoporotic compression fractures, spinal stenosis, ankylosing spondylitis, and septic diskitis. Conservative management is effective in the majority of cases of mechanical low back pain. This chapter will provide the practitioner a practical guide to the evaluation of low back pain.

FUNCTIONAL ANATOMY

The lumbar spine comprises functional elements including the vertebral bodies, lumbar discs, facet joints, nerve roots, and adjacent soft tissues. Practically, distinguishing among these various elements to determine the cause of low back pain is difficult in most cases. Nevertheless, the practitioner should be familiar with the various anatomic structures and their functional significance, and should understand the conditions unique to these various elements.

The intervertebral disc (Fig. 5.1.) and vertebral bodies together provide the bulk of the supporting structure of the spine. The interconnecting ligaments, facets, and paraspinal muscles provide additional stability.

The intervertebral disc is composed of a central nucleus of gelatinous material known as the nucleus pulposus. This nucleus area is highly enriched in proteoglycans. It is surrounded by the annular collagen rings of the annulus fibrosus, which impart torsional strength. Approximately 70% of the disc matrix is water. With aging, progressive desiccation and degeneration of the disc result, producing secondary disc-space narrowing. Desiccation also may predispose to disc protrusion and herniation resulting in nerve root compression or sciatica, which most commonly is the result of lateral protrusion of the disc. Central disc herniation in the lumbar spine is relatively infrequent and produces the characteristic symptoms of cauda equina syndrome due to direct compression of multiple sacral nerve roots.

The apophyseal or facet joints connect adjacent neural arches and facilitate flexion, extension, and, to a limited extent, rotation of the lumbar spine. These joints have a capsule and synovium, and they contain synovial fluid. Loss of disc height through degeneration with aging or

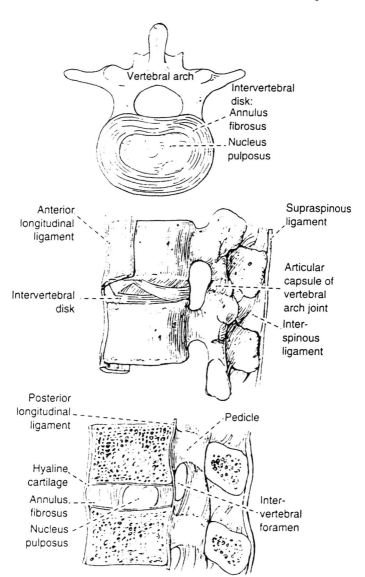

Figure 5.1 Joints and ligaments of the vertebrae.

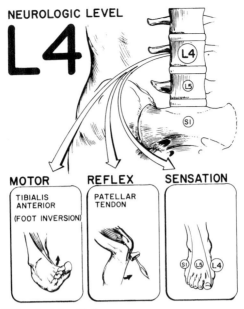

Figure 5.2 Neurologic level L-4.

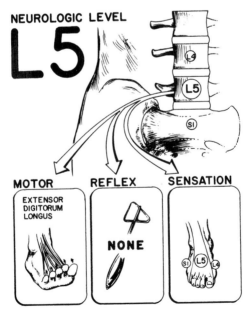

Figure 5.3 Neurologic level L-5.

trauma may lead to secondary degenerative changes in the articular cartilage of the facet joints, leading to osteoarthritis.

The nerve roots of the lumbar spine emerge from the conus of the chord located at the L-1 level, traveling downward almost vertically to exit through the corresponding vertebral body (Fig. 5.2). Because of this configuration, the exiting nerve root at each level is most susceptible to the disc immediately above where it passes under the pedicle. Therefore, for example, the L-5 root is most susceptible to compression by the L-4 disc (Fig. 5.3).

DIFFERENTIAL DIAGNOSIS

Most causes of low back pain are the result of biomechanical conditions (approximately 90%) (Table 5.1), including structural spine abnormalities, muscular conditions, and degenerative conditions. In general, distinguishing between biomechanical causes for most patients is difficult at best. Other medical conditions, such as vertebral fractures, inflammatory disorders, referred pain from other anatomic locations, and psychiatric conditions, account for the remainder (Table 5.1). Fac-

Table 5.1   Classification of Low Back Pain

Biomechanical (90%)	Medical (10%)
Structural spine abnormalities	**Trauma**
Kyphosis	Vertebral fracture
Scoliosis	Occupational factors
Muscular/ligamentous conditions	**Inflammatory**
Muscle spasm, atrophy	Infection
Degenerative disorders	Neoplasm
Intervertebral disc disease	Spondyloarthropathy
Facet osteoarthritis	**Metabolic conditions**
Spinal stenosis	Osteoporosis
Spondylolithesis	Osteomalacia
	Referred pain
	Abdominal aneurysm
	Retroperitoneal lesion
	Pyelonephritis
	Pancreatic disease
	Prostatitis
	Psychogenic
	Depression
	Fibromyalgia

Table 5.2   Historical Clues for Nonmechanical or Medical Causes of Low Back Pain

Weight loss
Night pain
Morning stiffness
Localized pain
Genitourinary/gastrointestinal symptoms

tors that should prompt consideration for these other medical conditions include weight loss, nocturnal pain, morning stiffness, localized pain, and associated gastrointestinal or genitourinary symptoms (Table 5.2).

EVALUATION

Key Decision Point: The initial evaluation of back pain should categorize it into one of four categories:

1. Mechanical
2. Inflammatory
3. Stenotic
4. Radicular

The evaluation of low back pain should include a careful history of the chronology, location, radiation, and factors aggravating and alleviating the low back pain. Additionally, the practitioner should inquire about symptoms that suggest medical or nonmechanical factors (Table 5.2). Both acute and chronic low back pain may be divided into acute and chronic forms, with chronic forms, particularly of the medical or nonmechanical causes, having a somewhat broader potential differential diagnosis. Mechanical back pain is suggested by pain that is precipitated by an injury, worsens with movement or activity, is relieved by rest, is not present at night, and is not associated with systemic symptoms such as fever or weight loss. Nonmechanical back pain is suggested by pain unrelated to (or in some cases relieved by) activity or movement, is present at night, or is associated with systemic symptoms such as fever or weight loss.

Key Decision Point: Magnetic resonance imaging generally is indicated if findings indicate radicular cause of back pain.

Low Back Pain
Chapter 5

Once mechanical back pain has been determined, the focus of the initial history should be to determine whether the pain is radicular or nonradicular (Fig. 5.4). Radicular pain is suggested by radiating pain into the lower extremity (generally extending below the knee), often accompanied by numbness or sensory loss in a peripheral dermatome distribution. The practitioner should attempt to determine whether there are objective signs correlating with radiculopathy on examination. These signs include (i) loss or decrease in knee or ankle deep tendon reflex; (ii) decreased sensation; (iii) positive straight leg raising test; (iv) weakness of great toe dorsiflexion (implicating S-1 root) (Figs. 5.2, 5.3, and 5.5) or ankle or knee extension; or (v) muscle atrophy. In general, symptoms of radiculopathy, when confirmed by objective signs on examination, should prompt further evaluation. The optimal and most cost-effective diagnostic test at this point is magnetic resonance imaging (MRI). If radiculopathy, typically the result of disc herniation, is confirmed by MRI, neurosurgical referral generally is indicated. For mechanical back pain without signs of radiculopathy, conservative management generally is indicated. One category of mechanical low back pain deserves special mention: spinal stenosis. Spinal stenosis is a condition in which there is narrowing of the canal

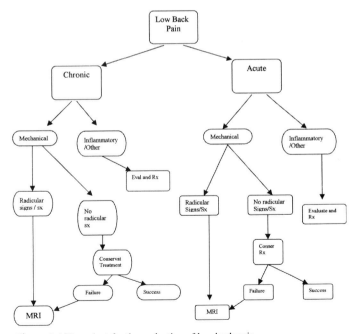

Figure 5.4 Flow chart for the evaluation of low back pain.

43

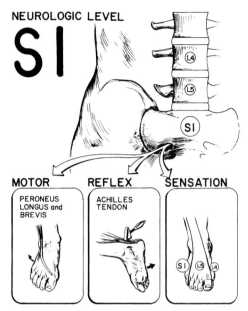

NEUROLOGIC LEVEL
S1

L4
L5
S1

| MOTOR | REFLEX | SENSATION |

PERONEUS LONGUS and BREVIS

ACHILLES TENDON

S1   L5   L4

Figure 5.5 Neurologic level S-1.

through which the lumbar nerve roots exit, typically producing neurogenic claudication. Patients with spinal stenosis frequently will describe low back or lower extremity pain that becomes progressively worse with ambulation and is relieved by rest or by leaning forward. Symptoms of weakness and paresthesias with progressive ambulation also are characteristic. This constellation of symptoms, especially with evidence of radiculopathy, should prompt additional imaging studies, generally an MRI, because this condition may be amenable to epidural corticosteroid injection and, in resistant cases, to surgical intervention.

> **Key Decision Point:** An evaluation that suggests spinal stenosis should prompt an MRI.

NONMECHANICAL OR MEDICAL BACK PAIN

For nonmechanical or medical back pain, the optimal evaluation is tailored to symptoms and physical examination. For example, if infection is suspected, blood cultures and additional imaging studies generally are indicated (this could include plain radiography, bone scanning, or MRI). If an osteoporotic fracture is suspected, plain radiography generally is sufficient. For suspected ankylosing spondylitis, the erythrocyte sedimentation rate and plain radiography, including the sacroiliac joints, is indicated. For suspected malignancy, the initial evaluation may include plain radiography, bone scans, or MRI.

MANAGEMENT

The management of low back pain depends on the results of the evaluation. Most patients with acute or chronic low back pain will have mechanical back pain without radicular symptoms or signs. Conservative therapy is indicated in these cases. In spinal stenosis, epidural corticosteroids frequently are helpful. Referral to an anesthesiologist or neurosurgeon is indicated if this treatment option is required. Optimal conservative therapy may include a brief period of rest, symptomatic medication therapy tailored to the individual, and physical modalities, such as stretching and flexibility exercises and walking.

6

Soft tissue disorders of the hip include **trochanteric bursitis, ischiogluteal bursitis, iliopsoas bursitis, osteitis pubis,** and **piriformis syndrome.** Of these, **trochanteric bursitis is the most common and appears to occur more frequently in women,** perhaps because of the broader female pelvis and increased resulting traction of the gluteals at their insertion on the greater trochanter (Fig. 6.1). Risk factors include overuse activities, such as jogging, and leg length discrepancies (with symptoms occurring on the side with the longer leg) (Fig. 6.2). The clinician should exclude true hip joint disease (which generally produces pain in the groin and is associated with abnormal passive range of motion in the joint), as well as referred pain from the abdomen (e.g., inguinal or femoral hernia) or (L3-4 disc herniation) lumbar spine.

> *Soft Tissue Disorders of the Hip and Pelvis*
> - Trochanteric bursitis
> - Ischiogluteal bursitis
> - Osteitis pubis
> - Piriformis syndrome

FUNCTIONAL ANATOMY

Hip joint movement is facilitated by several powerful muscle groups. Flexion is accomplished chiefly by the iliopsoas, with accessory function of the rectus femoris, pectineus, sartorius, and adductor longus. Extension is accomplished principally by the gluteus maximus and the hamstrings, with accessory function by the ischial head of the adductor magnus. Abduction is accomplished primarily by the gluteus medius, with the addition of the gluteus minimus. Adduction is accomplished primarily by the adductor magnus, with accessory function by the adductor longus, adductor brevis, pectineus, and gracilis. External rotation is accomplished by the gluteus maximus, quadratus femoris, and piriformis, with accessory function by the sartorius and gracilis. Internal rotation is accomplished by the gluteus minimus, with accessory function by the gluteus medius, adductor longus, adductor brevis, adductor magnus, pectineus, iliacus, and psoas. Normal hip range of motion varies with the manner in which it is examined. With the knee in flexion, the hip can be flexed to 120 degrees. With the knee extended, the hip can be flexed to only approximately 90 degrees, being limited by the pull of the hamstrings. Internal rotation is normally to 40 degrees, with external rotation to 45 degrees. Abduction is normally to 45 degrees and adduction to 20 to 30 degrees.

Hip Pain

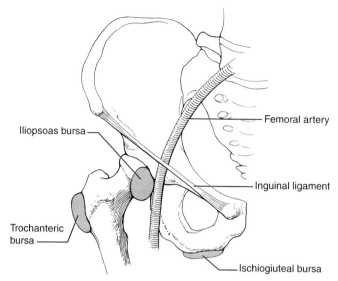

Femoral artery

Iliopsoas bursa

Inguinal ligament

Trochanteric bursa

Ischiogiuteal bursa

Figure 6.1 Bursae of the hip joint.

The normal gait cycle involves two basic phases: the stance phase and the swing phase (Fig. 6.3). The stance phase begins with heel contact. Full weight bearing begins with forefoot contact and ends with heel lift. The stance phase then ends with lift off and starts the swing phase. The swing phase then continues until heel contact and the cycle repeats. Under normal conditions, the stance phase comprises approximately 65% of the gait cycle, whereas the swing phase comprises approximately 45%. Hip disorders may cause the patient to walk with a shortened stance phase or with an antalgic gait, because he or she will try to minimize the time spent on full weight bearing. Chronic hip disorders frequently produce weakness of the gluteus medius or a Trendelenberg gait. Here hip abduction is impaired, and the pelvis on the opposite side drops during the stance phase. The body leans toward the diseased side when weight bearing is on the diseased hip.

Referred pain from the lumbar spine frequently complicates evaluation of hip pain. L4-5 radiculopathy, or occasionally L5-S1 radiculopathy in particular, may produce radiating symptoms to the lateral hip. The clinician should perform careful examination of motor and sensory systems, as well as reflexes of the lower extremity in the patient with hip pain. L4-5 radiculopathy may produce sensory loss of the medial lower leg, motor weakness of the anterior tibialis, and loss of the patellar reflex. L5-S1 radiculopathy may produce sensory loss of the lateral lower leg and foot, motor weakness of the extensor hallucis longus, and loss of the Achilles reflex.

Hip Pain

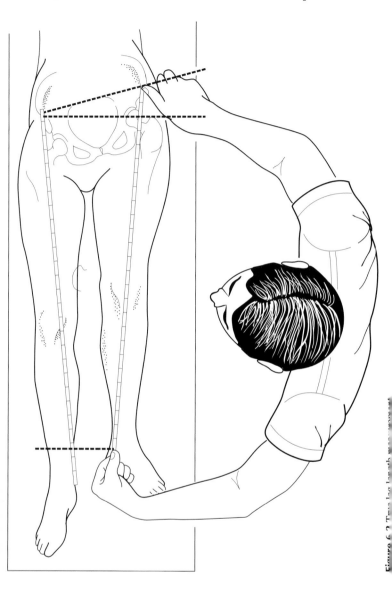

Figure 6-2 True leg length measurement

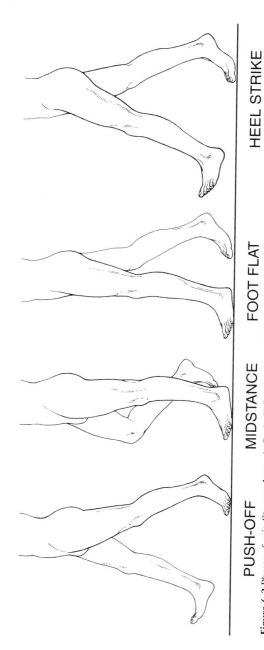

Figure 6.3 Phases of gait. **Stance phase. A:** Pushoff. **B:** Midstance. **C:** Foot flat. **D:** Heel strike.

PUSH-OFF   MIDSTANCE   FOOT FLAT   HEEL STRIKE

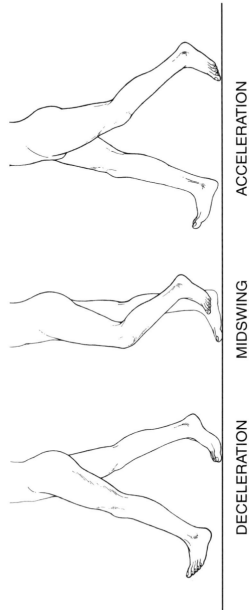

Figure 6.3 *(Continued)* Phases of gait. **Swing phase. A:** Deceleration. **B:** Midswing. **C:** Acceleration.

Hip Pain

DIFFERENTIAL DIAGNOSIS OF TROCHANTERIC BURSITIS

There are three bursae in the greater trochanteric region of the hip. The most important clinically and the largest is the gluteus maximus bursa, which separates the fibers of the gluteus maximus from the greater trochanter. The two other bursae lie between the gluteus medius and greater trochanter and the gluteus minimus and greater trochanter, respectively. Patients with trochanteric bursitis present with a deep, aching pain over the lateral upper thigh. The pain often is intensified by walking and may be worse at night, especially when the patient is lying on the affected side. The course is variable, with an acute phase lasting several days followed by gradual improvement and resolution over a period of days or weeks. In some cases, the course may be quite protracted, with symptoms persisting for months. The diagnosis is confirmed with palpation of the posterior aspect of the greater trochanter, which elicits local tenderness in this area. Resisted abduction of hip on the affected side also may be painful (Fig. 6.4).

The etiology of trochanteric bursitis is unknown; however, potential risk factors include local trauma, overuse activities, such as jogging, and leg length discrepancies (primarily on the side with the longer leg). These factors are believed to lead to increased tension of the gluteus maximus on the iliotibial band and produce bursal inflammation. The differential diagnosis of trochanteric bursitis includes lumbar radiculopathy (particularly the L-1 and L-2 nerve roots), meralgia paresthet-

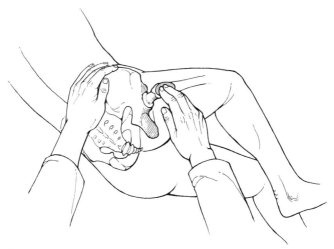

Figure 6.4 Trochanteric bursa. Trochanteric pain may be confused with sciatic pain.

ica (entrapment of the lateral cutaneous nerve of the thigh as it passes under the inguinal ligament), true hip joint disease, and intraabdominal pathology. These potentially confounding conditions generally can be excluded by careful history and physical examination.

Treatment of trochanteric bursitis is best accomplished by avoiding aggravating activity and local injection of a long-acting corticosteroid preparation. Referral to physical therapy in resistant cases may be helpful, particularly for exercises to stretch the iliotibial band.

ISCHIOGLUTEAL BURSITIS

The **ischiogluteal bursa** lies over the ischial tuberosity and facilitates gliding of the gluteus maximus muscle over the tuberosity. In the sitting position, the gluteus maximus slides superiorly, exposing the ischial tuberosity to potential friction.

Prolonged sitting on hard surfaces or repeated leg flexion and extension in the sitting position may predispose to repeated friction on the ischiogluteal bursa and lead to bursitis, also known as "weavers bottom." Rarely, the ischiogluteal bursa may become infected. The diagnosis is made by the characteristic history and by eliciting tenderness on palpation of the ischial tuberosity, with the patient lying supine and with the hip and knee flexed (Fig. 6.5). Treatment consists of using a cushioning "doughnut" seat and performing trunk and

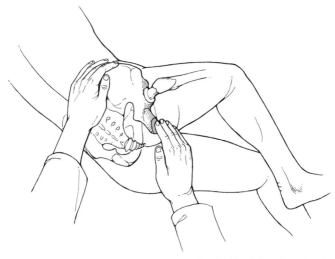

Figure 6.5 Ischiogluteal bursitis is easily confused with sciatic pain, unless the structures are isolated and the precise area of pain identified.

knee-to-chest stretching exercises while lying on the cushion. A local injection of corticosteroid is useful in refractory cases, although care should be taken to avoid the sciatic nerve, which lies just lateral to the ischiogluteal bursa.

ILIOPSOAS BURSITIS

The **iliopsoas bursa** (also called the iliopectineal bursa) lies over the anterior surface of the hip joint under the iliopsoas muscle and between the hip joint capsule. In most cases of reported iliopsoas, bursitis communication between the hip joint and the bursa occurs, either due to preexisting communication (which occurs in approximately 15% to 20% of normals) and associated excessive synovial fluid accumulation or to rupture of the hip joint capsule. The condition has been described in association with a number of hip disorders, including osteoarthritis, rheumatoid arthritis, synovial chrondromatosis, pigmented villonodular synovitis, osteonecrosis, and septic arthritis. Typically, patients present with an inguinal mass that may be painful and may be associated with secondary femoral vein obstruction or femoral nerve compression. Computerized tomography or magnetic resonance imaging are considered the optimal imaging methods to diagnose iliopsoas bursitis. Treatment of the underlying hip disorder generally is sufficient, although surgical excision sometimes is required.

OSTEITIS PUBIS (PUBIC SYMPHYSITIS)

Occasionally, **inflammation of the pubic symphysis** produces hip and groin pain with weight bearing. Pain typically is bilateral, but occasionally it may be more unilateral. This inflammatory lesion may be the result of chronic, repetitive stress, such as from running, from trauma, or in association with systemic inflammatory arthropathies. Examination shows localized, typically exquisite tenderness over the mons pubis. The x-ray films often show widening and erosions of the pubic symphysis. Initial treatment should involve local heat, antiinflammatory medications, and avoidance of prolonged weight bearing. In resistant or refractory cases, local injection of corticosteroid directly into the symphysis pubis occasionally is necessary and usually results in complete relief.

PIRIFORMIS SYNDROME

The piriformis muscle is an abductor and external rotator of the hip that occupies the greater sciatic foramen. Inflammation of the piriformis muscle insertion produces pain in the region of the sacroiliac joint often extending into the buttock, producing pain with ambulation. The

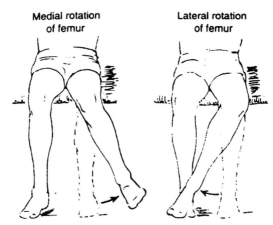

Figure 6.6 Medial and lateral rotation of the femur with the subject sitting, requiring the hips to be flexed. Medial and lateral rotation should be tested similarly with the hip extended, when the subject is lying prone with knees flexed 90 degrees. (Courtesy of Dr. D. Kay Clawson.)

history frequently includes trauma to the sacroiliac or gluteal region. Examination discloses pain and often weakness on resisted abduction and external rotation of the thigh (Fig. 6.6). Straight leg raising frequently is positive, but other neurologic signs, such as reduced or absent reflexes, lower extremity weakness, or sensory loss, are not present. Treatment includes stretching exercises, antiinflammatory medication, and, in resistant cases, local injection of corticosteroids.

7 ↪ Knee Pain

Many soft tissue disorders affect the knee joint, including the **bursitis syndromes** (involving the prepatellae and infrapatellae bursa, anserine bursa, gastrocnemius-semimembranous or popliteal bursa), iliotibial band syndrome, and a variety of **internal derangements within the joint** itself, such as tears of the meniscal cartilage or the collateral or cruciate ligaments. In additional, several syndromes involving the knee and its associated structures appear to occur primarily among adolescents. These include **Osgood-Schlatter disease** and **Sinding-Larsen-Johansson disease.** The most common cause of nonarticular knee pain is patellofemoral pain syndrome, formerly called chrondromalacia patellae. It appears to afflict primarily younger adults and is believed to result from abnormal patella tracking and/or repetitive microtrauma to the patella. When evaluating the painful knee, the clinician should remember that **significant mechanical derangement of the knee may occur in the absence of obvious trauma,** and this seems to be especially true of meniscal cartilage in the elderly, in whom preexisting degenerative disease may predispose to injury with normal daily activity.

Soft Tissue Disorders of the Knee

- Knee pain syndromes of adolescence
- Prepatellar bursitis
- Infrapatellar bursitis
- Anserine bursitis
- Gastrocnemius-semimembranous bursitis
- Iliotibial band syndrome
- Pelligrini-Stieda disease
- Plica syndrome
- Internal derangements
- Patellofemoral syndrome

FUNCTIONAL ANATOMY

The knee is the most complex and the largest joint in the human body (Fig. 7.1). It is a modified hinge joint with three compartments: the medial and lateral tibiofemoral compartments and the patellofemoral compartment. The knee is not a simple hinge joint, as it is capable of flexion, extension, and rotation. The latter movement occurs as the knee approaches full extension due to the shape of the joint surfaces and ligament tension, which causes internal rotation of the femur—the so-called "screwed-home position." Stability is pro-

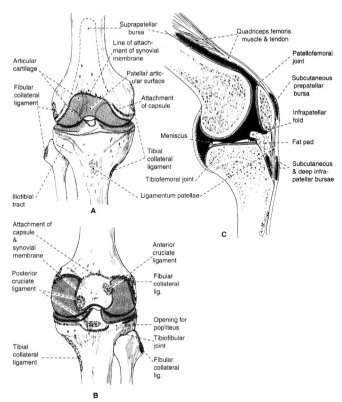

Figure 7.1 Anatomy of the knee joint showing the attachments of the capsule, synovial membrane, ligaments, and menisci. **A:** Anterior view. **B:** Posterior view. **C:** Sagittal section cut to one side of the midline. Cavities filled with synovial fluid are shown in *black* in (**C**).

vided by the cruciate ligaments and menisci and the capsule with its associated capsular ligaments.

The menisci or semilunar cartilages are crescent-shaped structures composed of fibrocartilage that transmit up to 70% of the force through the tibiotalar joint and have a lubricating role (Fig. 7.2). They are predominately avascular, although the peripheral 10% to 30% and the anterior and posterior horns receive blood supply from the geniculate vessels and, therefore, they have the capability for repair. The remainder of the menisci receive nutrients passively from the synovial fluid and have little capacity for repair. The anterior and posterior cru-

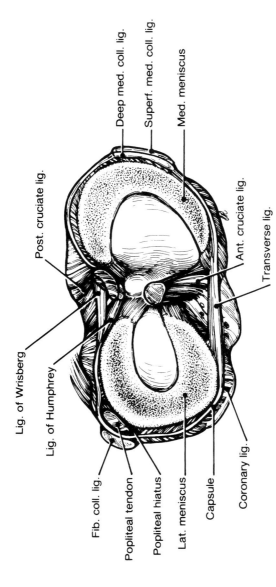

Figure 7.2 Medial and lateral menisci with their associated intermeniscal ligaments. (From Scott WN. *Ligament and extensor mechanism injuries of the knee: diagnosis and treatment*. St. Louis: Mosby-Year Book, 1991, with permission.)

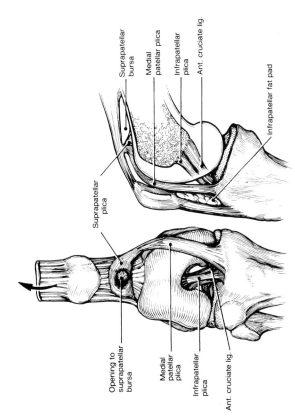

Figure 7.3 Intraarticular plicae of the knee. (From Scott WN. *Arthroscopy of the knee.* Philadelphia: WB Saunders, 1990, with permission.)

ciate ligaments together with the medial and lateral collateral ligaments are accessory ligaments of the capsule of the knee (Fig. 7.3). The anterior and posterior cruciate ligaments cross each other within the joint and are formed by twisting ropelike fibers of collagen of different lengths. The cruciate ligaments are the principal knee stabilizers in the anteroposterior plane, with the anterior cruciate preventing anterior slippage of the femur relative to the tibia and the posterior cruciate preventing posterior slippage. The cruciates also provide rotational stability. The collateral ligaments provide medial and lateral stability. The iliotibial band is a fascial band connecting the ilium with the lateral tibia. It contributes to the lateral stability of the knee (Fig. 7.4).

The patella is the largest sesamoid bone in the human body, and its undersurface possesses the thickest articular cartilage. The primary function of the patella is to increase the lever arm of the quadriceps. The stability of the patella is provided statically by the

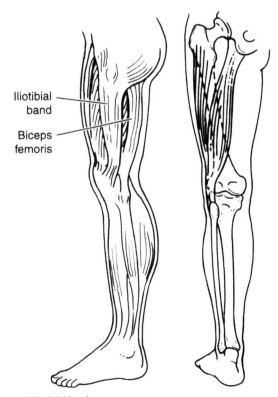

Iliotibial band

Biceps femoris

Figure 7.4 Iliotibial band.

bony interface between the trochlea of the femur and the undersurface of the patella. Dynamic stability is provided predominately by the extensor mechanism. There is considerable variation in the articular anatomy of the patella. The most common shape is a relatively larger lateral facet when compared to the medial facet. The shape of the femoral trochlea also varies considerably: it may be shallow and broad, deeply V shaped, or between these extremes. The quadriceps mechanism and its attachment to the knee is complex. Most anterior is the rectus femoris, which inserts anteriorly and most superficially to the patella. Medially, the vastus medialis inserts obliquely at an an-

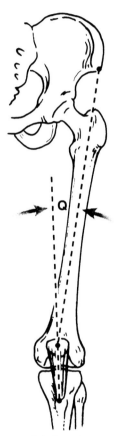

Figure 7.5 "Q" or quadriceps angle is formed by the intersection of the lines between the anterior superior iliac spine and the midportion of the patella and the tibial tubercle. It is the angle formed by the quadriceps muscle and the patellar tendon.

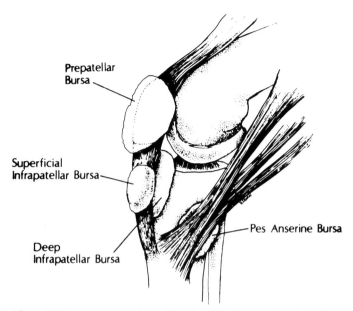

Figure 7.6 Bursae around the knee. (From Insall JN. *Surgery of the knee*. New York: Churchill Livingstone, 1984, with permission.)

gle of 60 to 70 degrees and provides dynamic medial stability for the patella, counteracting the lateral dynamic force on the patella imposed by the majority of the quadriceps mechanism, which is a consequence of the normal slight varus angulation of the lower leg in relation to the femur. Patellar tracking is influenced by the direction of pull of the quadriceps and the position of attachment of the patellar tendon into the tibial tubercle. This relationship is expressed by the **patella "Q" angle,** which is the angle formed by a line between the center of the patella extending proximally to the anterosuperior iliac spine and extending distally to the center of the tibial tubercle (Fig. 7.5). The normal Q angle is 10 degrees for men and 15 degrees for women. Femoral neck anteversion and external tibial torsion increases the Q angle, whereas femoral neck retroversion and internal tibial torsion decreases the Q angle. An excessive Q angle may predispose to patella subluxation or dislocation, because as the Q angle increases, the patella tends to track more laterally.

There are a number of bursae surrounding the knee joint (Fig. 7.6). Anteriorly is the subcutaneous, prepatellar bursa, which lies over the lower pole of the patella. Inferiorly are the infrapatellar bursae: the superficial infrapatellar bursa, which lies over the patella tendon and the tibial tubercle, and the deep infrapatellar bursa, which lies between the patellar tendon and the proximal tibia. Medial and inferior to the joint is the pes anserine bursa, which lies between the medial collateral ligament and the insertion of the adductor muscles of the thigh: the sartorius, gracilis, and semitendinosus. Posteriorly is the gastrocnemius-semimembranous bursa, which is a complex structure composed of three components: a base that is located under the capsular insertion of the gastrocnemius muscle, the medial extent between the heads of the gastrocnemius and the semimembranosus muscle, and a small subfascial extension. In more than 50% of individuals over 50 years of age, there is communication between the gastrocnemius-semimembranous bursa and the knee joint. When a communication exists, synovial fluid from any etiology may enter the bursa. If a large volume of synovial fluid suddenly expands into the gastrocnemius-semimembranous bursa, it may bulge into the popliteal fossa or it may rupture into the calf, producing the so-called "ruptured Baker's cyst" or pseudothrombophlebitis.

DIFFERENTIAL DIAGNOSIS

Knee Pain Syndromes of Adolescence

A variety of **knee pain syndromes occur in the adolescent** (10 to 18 years of age) and are unique to this age group. **Osgood-Schlatter disease** is one such condition that generally presents with activity-related pain around the tibial tubercle (Fig. 7.7). This condition is believed to result from submaximal, repetitive tensile stresses acting on the immature junction of the patellar ligament, tibial tubercle, and tibia, causing mild avulsion injury followed by attempts at osseous repair with proliferation of cartilage and bone. Pain generally is intermittent and increases with activities, especially those that require kneeling, squatting, or repeated jumping. An increased Q angle also has been associated with Osgood-Schlatter disease. Physical examination is notable for swelling and prominence of the tibial tubercle with local tenderness. In approximately 50% of cases, a discrete ossicle is noted at the tibial tubercle. Radiographs of the knee may be useful to exclude tumors and infection. Treatment with ice, antiinflammatory agents, an appropriately contoured knee pad, and maintenance of hamstring and quadriceps flexibility usually are sufficient to control symptoms that may take up to 12 months to resolve. Progressive or disabling symptoms may require a course of immobilization for 7 to 10 days.

Sinding-Larsen-Johansson disease is another cause of anterior knee pain in the adolescent and is similar to Osgood-Schlatter disease, except that tenderness is localized to the inferior pole of the patella or occasionally at the junction of the quadriceps tendon and the patella. This condition is believed to be the result of persistent traction at the cartilaginous junction of the patella and the patella ligament. Radiographs may show ossification at the junction of the patella and the ligament. The treatment program outlined for Osgood-Schlatter disease generally is successful in the management of Sinding-Larsen-Johansson disease.

PREPATELLAR BURSITIS

Prepatellar bursitis presents as painful, red swelling anterior to the knee cap and is seen most often in people who spend a lot of time kneeling, i.e., roofers and carpet fitters. Active knee extension usually is quite painful, although passive knee flexion usually is only minimally limited. **Infection and gout should be excluded** by aspirating any bursal fluid.

> **Key Decision Point:** Detection of bursal fluid or fluctulance about the knee (with the exception of a Baker's cyst, for which the knee proper should be aspirated) should lead to aspiration of the bursa. The bursal fluid should be cultured and examined for crystals.

In most cases, rest and avoiding sustained kneeling result in resolution. Septic bursitis usually is due to *Staphylococcus aureus* and requires antibiotic therapy as well as repeated drainage if fluid reaccumulates. Rarely, recurrent episodes of inflammation require surgical excision of the bursa.

INFRAPATELLAR BURSITIS

The deep **infrapatellar bursa** lies between the upper portion of the tibial tuberosity and patellar ligament. It is separated from the knee joint synovium by a fat pad (Fig. 7.7). Infrapatellar bursitis presents in a similar fashion as prepatellar bursitis, although the location of swelling and tenderness is in the soft tissues on either side of the patellar ligament just proximal to its insertion on the tibial tubercle. As a result, inflammation in this bursa may be more difficult to detect than in a subcutaneous bursa. The risk factors for development of infrapatellar bursitis are the same as for prepatellar bursitis.

ANSERINE BURSITIS

The anserine bursa lies under and about the pes anserinus, the insertion of the thigh adductor complex, which consists of the sartorius, gracilis, and semitendinosus muscles. It is located about 5 cm below the medial aspect of the joint space. Rarely, fluid distention of the bursa has been reported. Another bursa, the subtendinea musculi sar-

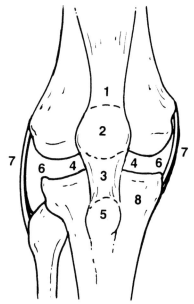

Figure 7.7 Palpation of pain in the knee. *1*, quadriceps tendinitis; *2*, prepatellar bursitis, patella pain; *3*, patella tendinitis; *4*, fat pad tenderness; *5*, Osgood-Schlatter disease (tibial tubercle pain); *6*, meniscus pain; *7*, collateral ligament pain; *8*, pes anserine tendinitis bursitis.

torii bursa, lies in this region, which is located approximately 0.5 to 1 cm cranial to the anserine bursa. Anserine bursitis is a term loosely applied to pain and associated local tenderness in this region, although "medial ligament" syndrome and pes anserinus tendinitis may be impossible to separate. Nocturnal pain often leading to use of a pillow between the knees is characteristic. Rarely, a palpable mass may be detected. Women seem more likely to develop anserine bursitis, perhaps because of broader pelvic area and greater angulation of the adductors at the knee joint, producing more tension on these attachments. Obesity and osteoarthritis of the knees appear to be additional predisposing factors. Optimal treatment includes the use of local corticosteroid injection mixed with local anesthetic.

GASTROCNEMIUS-SEMIMEMBRANOUS BURSITIS (BAKER'S CYST)

Any cause of synovitis in the knee can lead to leakage into the popliteal space when a communication exists with the gastrocnemius-semimembranous bursa. A communication between the gastrocnemius-semimembranous bursa and the anterior knee joint occurs in 40% of normal adults. Symptoms consist of fullness and tightness in the popliteal space that increases with walking. A **Baker's cyst** can be detected clinically by palpation of fullness in the medial third of popliteal fossa, although there is wide variation in the size of Baker's cysts, ranging from popliteal cysts to large calf cysts. Baker's cysts become softer with semiflexion and harder with extension of the knee (Foucher's sign). Knee effusions generally are present, although they may be small and often are overlooked. Baker's cysts may dissect into the muscles of calf simulating thrombophlebitis. The presence of crescentic bruising beneath the medial malleolus, the "hemorrhagic crescent sign," is believed to be a useful clinical clue to the presence of popliteal cyst rupture or calf hematoma. **Rupture of a Baker's cyst should be confirmed by Doppler ultrasound, which also can exclude thrombophlebitis of the popliteal vein.** To confirm a ruptured Baker's cyst, the ultrasonographer's attention must be directed to the soft tissue planes of the calf where dissecting fluid generally is seen. Rarely, rupture of a Baker's cyst causes associated thrombophlebitis or compressive neuropathy due to extensive venous or neural compression.

Treatment of an intact or ruptured Baker's cyst requires treating the cause of excess or abnormal synovial fluid production in the knee. Optimal management includes aspiration of the knee joint, with synovial fluid analysis and culture. Direct posterior aspiration of the Baker's cyst should not be performed because of the close proximity of neurovascular structures. In noninfectious synovitis of the knee, intraarticular instillation of corticosteroid is an effective treatment.

ILIOTIBIAL BAND SYNDROME (RUNNER'S KNEE)

The **iliotibial band** is a fascial band connecting the ilium with the lateral tibia, connecting to the tensor fasciae latae and the gluteus maximus. Repetitive flexion and extension, particularly with high-intensity running, can lead to inflammation of the iliotibial band or its associated bursa overlying the lateral femoral condyle. Excessive foot pronation resulting in tightening of the iliotibial band and increased friction across the femoral epicondyle also has been proposed as a cause of iliotibial band syndrome. Examination reveals tenderness localized to the lateral femoral condyle approximately 2 cm above the joint line, pain with weight bearing on the knee flexed 30 to 40 degrees, and a positive **Ober test** (the patient lies on his or her side with the lower leg flexed to eliminate lordosis of the lumbar spine, the knee of the upper leg is flexed to 90 degrees, and the thigh is abducted and extended; a positive test occurs when the hip remains abducted when the examiner's supporting hand is removed) (Fig. 7.8). Treatment consists of rest, locally applied heat, and orthotics when excessive foot pronation is present. Occasionally, a local injection of

Knee Pain

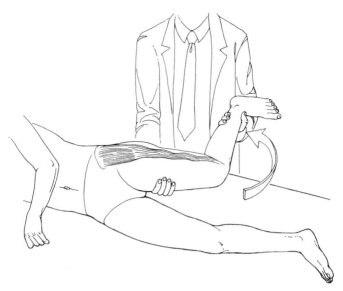

7.8A

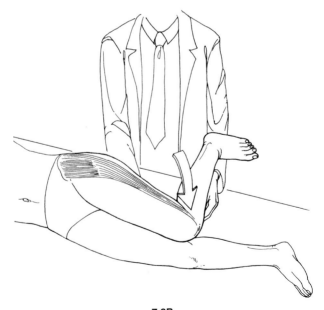

7.8B

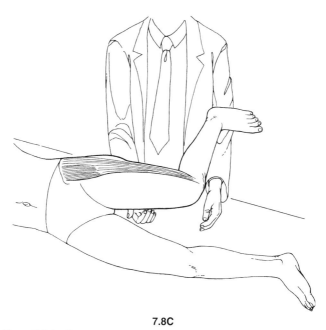

7.8C

Figure 7.8 A: Ober test to determine contraction of the fascia lata. **B:** Negative Ober. **C:** Positive Ober.

corticosteroid into the painful area is required. Partial resection of the iliotibial band over the lateral femoral condyle is reserved for the most resistant cases.

PELLIGRINI-STIEDA DISEASE

This condition results from **calcification of a hematoma at the femoral insertion of the medial collateral ligament following injury.** Examination reveals local tenderness and pain with application of valgus stress to the knee. Radiographs show characteristic calcification of the insertion of the medial collateral ligament. The condition usually is self-limited. Treatment consists of rest, nonsteroidal antiinflammatory agents, and occasionally local corticosteroid injection.

PLICA SYNDROME

Synovial plica are normal folds of the synovium that are remnants of the embryonic development of the synovial sac (Fig. 7.3). They are found in approximately 50% of cadaveric knees. With the advent of arthroscopy and direct visualization of these structures, they have been implicated in previously undiagnosed knee symptoms. Pathologic plica appear to result by two mechanisms: (i) direct trauma with resultant hemorrhage, edema, and progressive fibrosis; and (ii) overuse often associated with minor irregularities in knee mechanics causing progressive inflammation with recurrent synovitis, edema, and fibrosis with resultant thickening of the plica that then irritates surrounding tissue. Patients with symptomatic plica in the knee complain of snapping or popping of the knee at particular degrees of flexion. Medial plica are implicated most often as a cause of knee symptoms, presumably occurring when the plica rubs across the femoral condyle. Examination often reveals tenderness at the joint line and the palpation of the plica, especially with the knee in 20 degrees of flexion. Most patients respond to a combination of quadriceps strengthening and flexibility exercises and antiinflammatory medication. Surgical resection sometimes is advocated but remains a controversial therapy.

INTERNAL DERANGEMENTS

Internal derangements of the knee refer to **disruption of the normal functioning of the ligaments and menisci.** Disruption of the ligaments is most **often the result of significant, often athletic trauma.** Acute meniscal injury in young adults is usually the result of a twisting force applied to the weight-bearing knee and results in a longitudinal tear, which, if it is large enough, may cause the knee to lock (a "bucket handle" tear). Degenerative tears are more frequent in older adults and typically consist of radial tears. Chronic tears of this nature may occur without obvious trauma, but generally are accompanied by symptoms of knee locking or giving way. Examination generally reveals pain with forced extension and generally normal or only mildly reduced flexion. **McMurray's test** (flexing and extending the knee while the tibia is internally and then externally rotated; a positive test is indicated by pain and/or an associated click) may be helpful if positive, but the test is relatively insensitive (Fig. 7.9).

In the United States, magnetic resonance imaging (MRI) is widely used to diagnose suspected meniscal tears and to help plan the therapeutic approach. Early studies with MRI suggest a relatively high rate of false-positive findings. With the current improvement in technology and experience, this appears to less of a problem, although there still may be substantial variation in accuracy among centers.

> **Key Decision Point:** Suspected mechanical derangement of the knee should prompt an MRI of the knee. Referral to an orthopedic surgeon is indicated if mechanical derangement is confirmed.

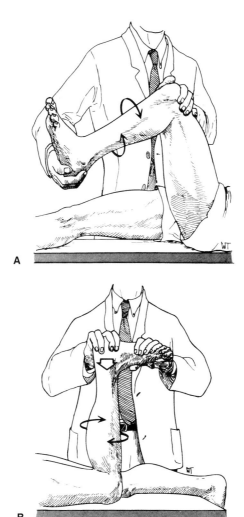

Figure 7.9 A: McMurray's test is performed with the knee flexed 90 degrees and slowly extended with an external rotation force. It might be positive for a posterior peripheral medial meniscus tear. (From Insall JN. *Surgery of the knee.* New York: Churchill Livingstone, 1984, with permission.) **B:** In the Apley test, the prone patient flexes the knee 90 degrees. The examiner compresses the joint while simultaneously rotating it. Meniscal pain often is discovered, yet this test is by no means pathognomonic of a meniscal tear.

Symptomatic peripheral tears (i.e., the outer one third) of the meniscus in the young adult generally are repaired because there is potential for healing. Partial meniscectomy is recommended if tears involve the avascular inner two thirds of the meniscus. Nonoperative treatment can be considered in the older patient with a degenerative meniscal tear, although arthroscopic resection may be required for persistent symptoms. Total meniscectomy generally is avoided because long-term follow-up studies demonstrated high rates of osteoarthritis following this procedure.

PATELLOFEMORAL PAIN SYNDROME

Chondromalacia patellae is a term that has been used synonymously with **patellofemoral pain.** Most authorities now urge that the term be abandoned in this setting, given the almost universal presence of asymptomatic cartilage changes on the medial facet of the patella and the observation via arthroscopy that most, if not many, individuals with anterior knee symptoms have normal articular surfaces. Chrondromalacia patellae now is recommended to connote gross pathologic observation made operatively or at autopsy. **Patellofemoral pain now is the recommended term applied to label ill-defined anterior knee pain.**

Patellofemoral pain syndrome is used most commonly to describe poorly localized anterior knee pain, frequently accompanied by the **"grab sign"** (patients cover the entire front of the knee with the hand when asked to localize the location of the discomfort). Pain frequently occurs after prolonged sitting with flexed knees, the so-called "theater" sign. Physical examination may reveal tenderness of the medical or lateral facets of the patella, pain with compression of the patella on the femoral condyle, or a patellar "shrug" sign (pain when pressure is applied to the patella while the patient contracts the quadriceps). An abnormally increased Q angle (greater than 15 degrees in males and greater than 20 degrees in females) appears to predispose to patellofemoral pain. The Q angle is easily measured by determining the angle formed between a line drawn from the anterior superior iliac spine to the midpoint of the patella and a line drawn from the tibial tubercle to the same point on the patella. Patellofemoral pain syndrome is believed to result either from anatomic abnormalities (such as anatomic misalignment of the patella tracking mechanism, quadriceps dysplasia, or patellofemoral ligament imbalance) or from repetitive microtrauma to the patella surface. Standard radiographs usually are not helpful in the evaluation of anterior knee pain, particularly for patellar tracking, because most tracking abnormalities occur during dynamic use. Nonoperative treatment of idiopathic anterior knee pain is successful in 75% to 90% of patients. Treatment modalities include avoidance of overuse, exercises, orthoses, and antiinflammatory medications.

8

↪ Foot and Ankle Pain

Soft tissue disorders of the foot and ankle are among the most common afflictions to affect humans and often result from ill-fitting footwear (e.g., high heels, excessively narrow toe box), overuse injuries (e.g., running), or abnormal biomechanical factors (e.g., excess pronation, flat feet), either alone or in combination. These conditions include Achilles tendinitis, retrocalcaneal bursitis, plantar fasciitis, metatarsalgia, Morton's or interdigital neuroma, and tarsal tunnel syndrome. **Middle-aged and older adults seem to be most prone to foot conditions,** probably because many of these conditions require years of weight-bearing stress to develop. Identification of these conditions and treatment directed at the underlying biomechanical precipitants generally result in significant symptomatic benefit.

Soft Tissue Disorders of the Foot

- Achilles tendinitis
- Retrocalcaneal bursitis
- Plantar fasciitis
- Metatarsalgia
- Morton's neuroma
- Tarsal tunnel syndrome

FUNCTIONAL ANATOMY

The foot is composed of 26 bones and 38 muscles, along with a variable number of sesamoids that are held together by 125 interconnecting ligaments, and must absorb up to six times the body weight with each step (Fig. 8.1). The foot usually is divided into three sections: the forefoot, the midfoot, and the hindfoot. The forefoot consists of the five metatarsals and is separated from the midfoot by the tarsometatarsal joint of Lisfranc. The midfoot contains the three cuneiforms, the navicular, and the cuboid, separated from the hindfoot by the transverse midtarsal joint. The hindfoot is composed of the calcaneus and the talus.

The ankle joint is composed of three articulations: the tibiotalar joint, the subtalar joint, and the talonavicular joint. The tibiotalar joint or "true" ankle joint is the result of the articulation of the dome of the talus, the roof or plafond of the distal tibia, and the distal tibiofibular joint. The joint is stabilized medially by the medial bony protrusion of the distal tibia, the medial malleolus, and the distal lateral fibula forming the lateral malleolus. Motion at the tibiotalar joint consists of 20 degrees of dorsiflexion and 50 degrees of plantar flexion. A com-

Foot and Ankle Pain

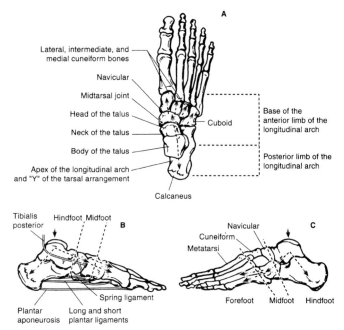

Figure 8.1 Tarsal bones and dispersion of weight throughout the foot. **A:** Superior view. **B:** Medial view. **C:** Lateral view.

plex set of ligaments additionally stabilizes the ankle. The deltoid ligament (composed of four ligaments: the posterior tibiotalar ligament, the tibiocalcaneal ligament, the tibionavicular ligament, and the anterior tibiotalar ligament) provides medial stability. The lateral collateral ligament (composed of the posterior talofibular ligament, the calcaneofibular ligament, and the anterior talofibular ligament) provides lateral stability (Fig. 8.2).

The **subtalar joint** is composed of the articulation of the calcaneus and the talus, is surrounded by its own distinct capsule, and does not articulate with other joints. The normal range of motion of the subtalar joint is 5 degrees of inversion and 5 degrees of eversion. The subtalar joint provides inversion and eversion of the heel and facilitates walking on uneven terrain. The transverse midtarsal joint of Chopart is composed of the talonavicular joint and the calcaneocuboid joint and permits multiaxial motion: inversion and eversion of the midfoot and forefoot and, to a lesser degree, dorsiflexion and plantar flexion and abduction and adduction. It is stabilized by the bifurcate ligament, which has two components: the calcaneonavicular segment and the calcaneocuboid component. The tarsometatarsal joint of Lisfranc is composed of the interconnected second through fifth tarsometatarsal joints. A complex set of ligaments on their dorsal and plantar aspects provide stability and consists of two principal components: the dorsal tarsometatarsal ligaments and the plantar tarsometatarsal ligaments.

The **metatarsophalangeal (MTP) joints** are analogous to the metacarpophalangeal joints of the hands and are stabilized by the deep transverse metatarsal ligament and the plantar ligaments. The first MTP joint plays a critical role in normal gait. Under most conditions, 65 to 75 degrees of dorsiflexion of the hallux on the first metatarsal is required for normal gait and for the hallux to function in propulsion. Disorders such as hallux valgus and hallux rigidus affect gait adversely by limiting dorsiflexion of the first MTP joint.

The **interphalangeal joints** of the toes are analogous to those of the hand and consist of hinge joints stabilized by collateral ligaments and a plantar capsular ligament with a fibrous plate. The plantar aponeurosis or plantar fasciae runs from the plantar aspect of the calcaneus to the region of the metatarsal heads. It is composed of two distinct layers, the superficial and deep. The superficial layer blends with subcutaneous tissue, whereas the deep layer joins the deep transverse metatarsal ligament and the flexor tendons.

Attached to the foot and ankle are the tendons of the extrinsic muscles, which form three compartments in the lower leg: the anterior compartment containing the dorsiflexors or extensors of the foot and ankle, the lateral compartment containing the peroneal muscles that act as plantar flexors and abductors, and the posterior compartment that con-

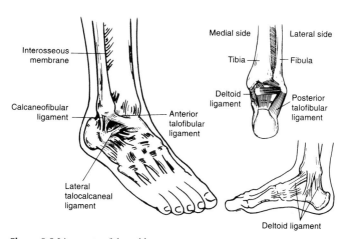

Figure 8.2 Ligaments of the ankle.

Foot and Ankle Pain

tains the plantar flexors. Posterior to the ankle is the Achilles tendon formed by the conjoined tendons of the gastrocnemius and the soleus muscles, which function to plantar flex the foot. Medially at the ankle is the tibialis posterior tendon complex, which is composed of the tendons of the flexor digitorum longus, the tibialis posterior, and the flexor hallucis longus, which pass underneath the flexor retinaculum posterior to the medial malleolus. Between the sheaths of the flexor digitorum longus and the flexor hallucis longus tendons lies the posterior tibial artery and nerve within the tarsal tunnel. Tenosynovitis of the tibialis posterior, flexor hallucis longus, or flexor digitorum longus tendons may produce functional compression of the posterior tibial nerve, producing tarsal tunnel syndrome. The tibialis posterior is the principal inverter of the foot and maintains the longitudinal arch by its insertion to the navicular and medial and intermediate cuneiforms and bases of the second, third, and forth metatarsals. Laterally at the ankle, passing under the superior and inferior peroneal retinacula, is the common sheath of the peroneus longus and brevis tendons, which are the principal everters and abductors of the foot. Anteriorly, the extrinsic extensor tendons of the foot (the extensor digitorum longus, the peroneus tertius, and the extensor hallucis longus tendons) within their tendon sheaths pass under the fibrous superior and inferior extensor retinacula.

There are several pertinent bursae of the foot and ankle. The retrocalcaneal bursa lies between the calcaneus anteriorly and the Achilles tendon posteriorly. This bursa has a synovial lining that abuts the Achilles fat pad. Anteriorly, the bursal wall is composed of fibrocartilage and posteriorly is contiguous with the Achilles tendon (Fig. 8.3). The bursa itself is horseshoe shaped, with the average length of the legs measuring 22 mm and a width of 4 mm. Between the skin and the Achilles tendon posteriorly is the subcutaneous calcaneal bursa. At the plantar aspect of the midcalcaneus is the subcalcaneal bursa.

DIFFERENTIAL DIAGNOSIS OF HEEL PAIN

Achilles Tendinitis

The most common causes of heel pain are Achilles tendinitis, retrocalcaneal bursitis, and plantar fasciitis. Achilles tendinitis generally is caused by repetitive trauma and microscopic tears of the tendon at its insertion on the calcaneus. Occasionally, Achilles tendinitis may be seen in patients with seronegative spondyloarthropathies without a history of overuse. The usual presentation is gradual onset of pain with foot pushoff. Physical examination reveals tenderness and occasional thickening of the tendon. Rest, antiinflammatory medication, a heel lift, gentle stretching exercises, and local heat application are effective treatment measures. The Achilles tendon is vulnerable to rupture in the

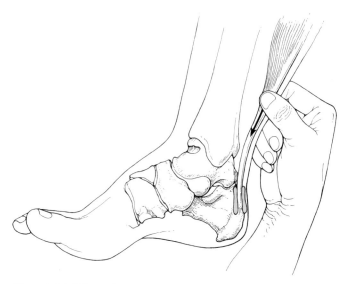

Figure 8.3 Achilles tendon.

elderly. In resistant cases, carefully applied local injection along the sides of the tendon can be attempted.

RETROCALCANEAL BURSITIS

The **retrocalcaneal bursa** resides between the Achilles tendon and a fat pad posterior to the talus (Fig. 8.4). Retrocalcaneal bursitis is associated with posterior heel pain that is made worse with passive dorsiflexion of the ankle that may be associated with tender swelling on both sides of the insertion of the tendon. Causes include repetitive trauma due to athletic activity, rheumatoid arthritis, and all of the seronegative spondyloarthropathies. Treatment is the same as for Achilles tendinitis, although cautious use of local corticosteroid injection may be necessary in resistant cases.

PLANTAR FASCIITIS

Plantar fasciitis is attributed to repetitive microtrauma to the attachment of the plantar fascia at the calcaneus producing periostitis and degenerative changes in the origin of the plantar fascia (Fig. 8.5). Localized pain with weight bearing on the undersurface of the heel is the typical presentation. Examination shows local tenderness over the an-

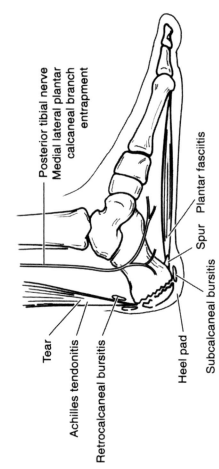

Figure 8.4 Sites and possible causes of heel pain.

Posterior tibial nerve
Medial lateral plantar calcaneal branch entrapment

Plantar fasciitis

Spur

Subcalcaneal bursitis

Heel pad

Retrocalcaneal bursitis

Achilles tendonitis

Tear

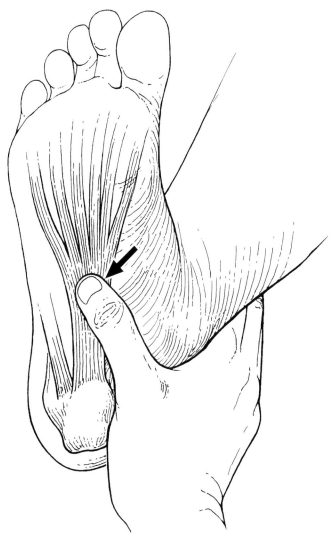

Figure 8.5 Plantar aponeurosis.

teromedial portion of the plantar surface of the calcaneus, with symptoms worsening on passive dorsiflexion of the toes. Radiographs may show a plantar calcaneal spur. Associated conditions include enthesopathy due to any of the seronegative spondyloarthropathies. Subcalcaneal or infracalcaneal bursitis may be difficult to distinguish from plantar fasciitis, although passive dorsiflexion of the toes does not increase symptoms. Treatment consists of a heel pad or cushion, rest, application of local heat, stretching exercises, and antiinflammatory agents. Nocturnal splinting to maintain passive stretching of the plantar fascia may help relieve morning pain and stiffness. Taping of the foot using the Low-Dye method also may be helpful. Local injection of corticosteroid at the insertion of the plantar fascia may be useful (Fig. 8.6). The vast majority of patients respond to these conservative measures. Surgical approaches, such as fasciotomy and spur excision, are infrequently required in resistant cases.

METATARSALGIA

Metatarsalgia is the symptom of pain across the plantar surface of one or more MTP joints and may be due to diverse causes, including muscle imbalance, fat pad atrophy, Morton's neuroma, hallux valgus, hallux rigidus, callosities, flat (pes planus) or cavus foot, arthritis of the MTP joints, intermetatarsophalangeal bursitis, tarsal tunnel syndrome, and arterial insufficiency. Symptomatic treatment (for patients with muscle imbalance and fat pad atrophy) includes the use of a metatarsal pad and flexion exercises. Arch supports are recommended for patients with flat or pronated feet.

HALLUX VALGUS AND RIGIDUS

Hallux valgus and **hallux rigidus** are common deformities of the great toe that produce pain in the first MTP joint. While these are technically not soft tissue, they are among the most common causes of foot pain. Hallux valgus may result from excessively narrow foot wear or high heels or from osteoarthritis of the first MTP joint. It often is associated with bursitis over the medial aspect of the MTP or bunion and, as a result of altered weight bearing, may result in secondary callosities under the second MTP joint and a hammer toe deformity of the second toe. Treatment consists of the use of accommodating footwear and bunion pad. Surgical correction may be required for resistant cases or marked deformities.

Hallux rigidus produces progressive pain and loss of motion in the first MTP joint. The causes are potentially multiple and include osteoarthritis of the first MTP and congenital deformities of the hallux. Conservative treatment is designed to reduce the need for first MTP dorsiflexion and consists of wide, stiff-soled shoes. Surgical proce-

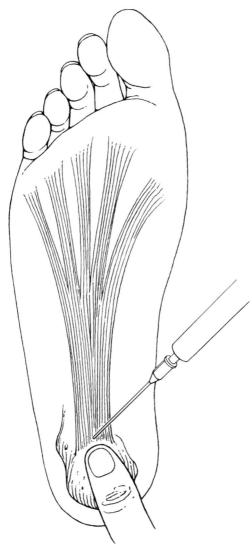

Figure 8.6 Local injection of corticosteroid at the insertion of the plantar fascia.

dures, such as bunionectomy, implant arthroplasties, and first MTP fusion, are advocated for severely affected patients.

MORTON'S NEUROMA

Morton's neuroma is a relatively common cause of foot pain and is caused by neurofibroma or perineural fibrosis of the large superficial branch of the external plantar nerve between the metatarsal heads (Fig. 8.7). The most common cause probably is repetitive microtrauma of the common digital nerve. Women seem to be affected more often than men, probably because of increased use of tight-fitting footwear. The typical presentation is paresthesias or dysesthesias in interdigital web spaces, particularly between the third and fourth interspaces. Pain is increased by weight bearing or with the use of tight-fitting footwear. Examination reveals interspace tenderness with palpation. The diagnosis may be confirmed with injection of 1% lidocaine into the interspace, which results in almost immediate relief in symptoms. Treatment consists of using footwear with low heels and wider widths. Local injection of corticosteroids or surgical resection may be required in resistant cases.

TARSAL TUNNEL SYNDROME

Tarsal tunnel syndrome most often refers to compression of the posterior tibial nerve as it courses around the medial malleolus with the posterior tibial artery and the tibialis posterior, flexor digitorum longus, and flexor hallucis tendons under the flexor retinaculum (Fig. 8.4). Tarsal tunnel syndrome has diverse potential etiologies, including mechanical factors such as excessive subtalar joint pronation, tenosynovitis of the tendons accompanying the posterior tibial nerve, synovitis of the ankle joint, and trauma. The typical presentation is with dysesthesias involving the plantar aspect of the foot, often more prominent at night. Examination reveals a **Tinel's sign** with percussion of the flexor retinaculum. Reduced vibratory sensation and decreased two-point discrimination may be present on the plantar aspect of the foot and toes. The diagnosis of tarsal tunnel syndrome may be confirmed by nerve conduction studies documenting delay in conduction of the posterior tibial nerve across the ankle. Magnetic resonance imaging may be useful in the evaluation of the relevant anatomic structures. Conservative treatment consists of local corticosteroid injection, use of nonsteroidal antiinflammatory drugs, and orthotic devices. Surgical decompression of the posterior tibial nerve is reserved for resistant cases.

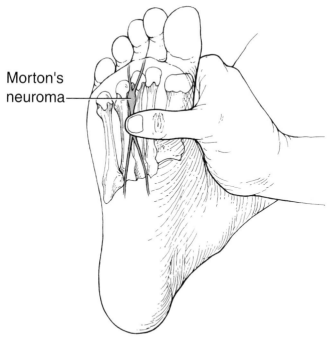

Morton's
neuroma

Figure 8.7 Morton's neuroma, a painful neuroma usually located between the third and fourth metatarsal heads.

9 ❧ Fibromyalgia

Fibromyalgia syndrome is a controversial chronic pain syndrome characterized by the clinical features of chronic, widespread musculoskeletal pain and diffuse soft tissue tenderness. Formerly known as fibrositis, the term fibromyalgia has become popular more recently in the absence of inflammatory signs. Although the pathophysiology of fibromyalgia remains unknown, the weight of evidence suggests that central or more specifically psychological factors play a prominent and probably crucial role. Convincing population-based evidence suggests that depression is the principal risk factor in the development of the syndrome. Neurochemical and neurohormonal abnormalities that have been observed thus far appear to be nonspecific and may overlap with, or are confounded by, similar findings observed in affective disorders. Ultimately, **fibromyalgia syndrome probably will defy the mind–body dualists, because it possesses features of both. Fibromyalgia syndrome at this time probably is best viewed within the context of the "affective spectrum." This spectrum includes panic disorder, irritable bowel syndrome, migraine, major depression, chronic fatigue syndrome, and fibromyalgia.**

The diagnosis of fibromyalgia has been facilitated by **classification criteria developed by the American College of Rheumatology.** These criteria, in turn, have enabled investigators to perform population-based studies that have further characterized the syndrome. In contrast to earlier clinic-based studies that were retrospective, population-based studies suggest that the association of fibromyalgia with affective disorders is constitutive rather than associative. The disorder has its peak prevalence in middle-aged and older women, with about a 10:1 female-to-male ratio. Long-term studies suggest that the condition persists over time, with about 15% of patients receiving disability payments for the condition. Symptoms of fibromyalgia commonly associated with chronic, widespread musculoskeletal pain include difficulty sleeping, fatigue, intermittent paresthesias, and symptoms of irritable bowel syndrome. Diffuse tenderness associated with fibromyalgia is exaggerated at the so-called tender point sites, which represent convenient locations to elicit a low pain threshold (Fig. 9.1).

ACR Classification Criteria for Fibromyalgia Syndrome

1. History of chronic widespread pain
Definition: Pain is considered widespread when present above and below the waist, on both sides of the body. Chronic is defined as longer than 3 months in duration.

Fibromyalgia

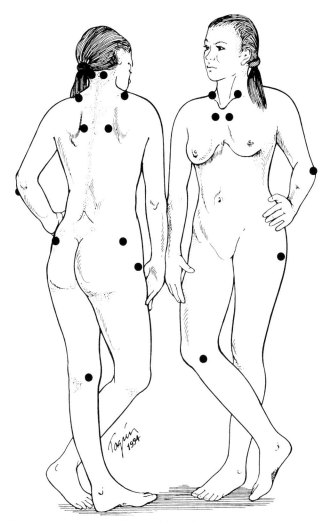

Chapter 9

Figure 9.1 Tender points in fibromyalgia syndrome.

> *ACR Classification Criteria for Fibromyalgia Syndrome*
> (Continued)
>
> **2. Pain in 11 of 18 tender points on digital palpation**
>   Occiput, low cervical, trapezius, supraspinatus,
>   second rib, lateral epicondyle, gluteal, greater
>   trochanter, knee
>   For classification purposes, patients are said to have
>   fibromyalgia if both criteria are satisfied.

DIFFERENTIAL DIAGNOSIS

Several conditions mimic the presentation of fibromyalgia, including hypothyroidism, early rheumatoid arthritis (RA), systemic lupus erythematosus (SLE), and polymyalgia rheumatica (PMR). Careful physical examination and selected laboratory tests usually will distinguish fibromyalgia from these inflammatory or metabolic conditions. Fibromyalgia is not associated with objective abnormalities on musculoskeletal examination, whereas early RA, SLE, or PMR typically shows abnormalities on joint examination. In addition, laboratory studies, especially acute phase reactants such as the erythrocyte sedimentation rate, are abnormally elevated in RA, SLE, and PMR, even when there are subtle abnormalities on joint examination.

> *Differential Diagnosis of Fibromyalgia*
>
> •Hypothyroidism
> •Early rheumatoid arthritis
> •Systemic lupus erythematosus
> •Polymyalgia rheumatica

EVALUATION

The onset of symptoms of fibromyalgia typically is insidious, although occasionally patients may attribute a precipitating event to the onset of symptoms. Patients typically complain of "pain all over" and "few or no days" without pain. There often is a prior history of depression or anxiety disorder. The examination shows normal joints and neuromuscular examination. Moderate pressure over muscles and tendon insertions, such as the midtrapezius, lateral and medial epicondyles, suboccipital insertion, rhomboids, greater trochanters, and anserine bursae, typically elicits marked bilateral tenderness with grimacing and/or withdrawal.

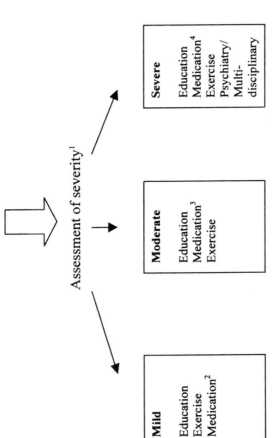

Diagnosis of Fibromyalgia

Assessment of severity[1]

Mild

Education
Exercise
Medication[2]

Moderate

Education
Medication[3]
Exercise

Severe

Education
Medication[4]
Exercise
Psychiatry/
Multi-
disciplinary

Figure 9.2 Management of fibromyalgia syndrome. *1.* Assessment of severity includes evaluation of pain, sleep, and fatigue symptoms, as well as functional impairment (for example, impact of symptoms on employment). *2.* Medication for mild symptoms might include only low-dose tricyclic. *3.* Medication for moderately severe symptoms might include the combination of a selective serotonin reuptake inhibitor with low-dose tricyclic. *4.* Medication regimen for severe symptoms initially would include that recommended for moderate symptoms, but may require revision in coordination with a psychiatrist.

MANAGEMENT

The treatment of fibromyalgia includes reassurance that the condition is not a progressive, crippling, or life-threatening entity. **A combination of treatment options that include medication and physical measures is helpful in most patients.** The severity of symptoms, and especially how they affect the functional status of the patient with fibromyalgia, is helpful to determine the approach to treatment (Fig. 9.2). Patients with relatively mild symptoms with little impact on physical function may not require medication. Medication shown to be helpful in short-term, double-blind, placebo-controlled trials include amitriptyline (Elavil) and cyclobenzaprine (Flexeril). Low doses of these medications (e.g., 10 to 30 mg of amitriptyline or 10 to 30 mg of cyclobenzaprine) are moderately effective and generally well tolerated. Recent studies have shown that newer antidepressants of the selective serotonin reuptake inhibitor class also are effective, particularly in combination with low doses of tricyclic agents. This approach should be considered for patients who are affected more severely. Corticosteroids and chronic use of narcotic analgesics are not indicated in the management of patients with fibromyalgia. Patients with fibromyalgia should be encouraged to take an active role in the management of their condition. If possible, they should begin a progressive, low-level aerobic exercise program to improve muscular fitness and sense of well-being. A combination approach is effective in alleviating symptoms in most patients, although a small minority of patients require more intensive treatment strategies, such as psychiatric or pain center referral.

Medications Useful in the Management of Fibromyalgia

Amitriptyline
Nortriptyline
Cyclobenzaprine
Fluoxetine
Paroxetine
Sertraline

---

10   ↳ Injection Techniques

Local injection is an integral component of the effective management of soft tissue disorders. Corticosteroids most commonly are injected into soft tissue structures either alone or sometimes in combination with an anesthetic agent. Common soft tissue disorders in which local injection is particularly effective include subacromial bursitis, bicipital tendinitis, digital stenosing tenosynovitis, carpal tunnel syndrome, de Quervain's tenosynovitis, trochanteric bursitis, anserine bursitis, and retrocalcaneal bursitis. **Aspiration of soft tissue structures occasionally is required for appropriate diagnosis (e.g., aspiration of a suspected septic olecranon bursa).**

CORTICOSTEROID PREPARATIONS

Corticosteroids administered via local injection generally are safe, effective, and well-tolerated. Their mode of action is presumed to be antiinflammatory. Minimal systemic absorption occurs with local injection, although occasionally poorly controlled diabetics experience a transient increase in blood sugar levels following local corticosteroid injection. Other systemic side effects of long-term oral or high-dose administration of corticosteroids, such as adrenal suppression, osteoporosis, myopathy, mental status changes, cushingoid appearance, fluid retention, hypertension, avascular necrosis, and increased risk of infection, generally are not seen. **More common problems with locally injected corticosteroids include postinjection pain** (may be due to a volume effect or to an inflammatory response to the steroid vehicle), **skin depigmentation or atrophy** (usually due to poor technique or excessive amount of corticosteroid), **and, rarely, tendon rupture** (usually due to injection directly into the tendon as opposed to the tendon sheath).

Corticosteroid preparations commonly used in soft tissue injections are listed with comparative concentrations in Table 10.1. Most practitioners seem to prefer either of two intermediate-acting corticosteroid preparations: triamcinolone or methylprednisolone. There is no evidence that one preparation is superior, but methylprednisolone possesses more concentration options. One may use relatively low concentrations for local superficial injection, such as for finger tendon sheaths, and relatively high concentrations for deeper injections, such as for subacromial bursa or trochanteric bursa. In general, the author prefers not to combine the corticosteroid with anesthetic, due to the increased volume effect, the short-lasting effect of the anesthetic, and the tendency to cause precipitation of the corticosteroid.

Injection Techniques

Table 10.1 Corticosteroid Preparations

Corticosteroid Preparation	Concentration
Short acting	
Hydrocortisone	25 mg/mL
Intermediate-acting	
Methylprednisolone (Depo-Medrol)	20–80 mg/mL
Triamcinolone acetonide (Kenalog)	10 mg/mL
Triamcinolone hexacetonide (Aristospan)	20 mg/mL
Long-acting	
Dexamethasone (Decadron)	4 mg/mL

STERILE TECHNIQUE

Only prepacked disposable needles and syringes should be used. Single-dose ampules of corticosteroid are preferable. Needles should be changed after drawing up the solution prior to injection. Gloves should be worn, but they need not be sterile. The site of injection can be marked with a retracted ballpoint pen and should be swabbed twice with an iodine-based solution and allowed to dry (a wet iodine-based surface may not be bacteria free). Local anesthetic with amyl nitrate spray then may be applied. The needle should not be touched during the procedure.

NEEDLES AND SYRINGES

Small-caliber needles are best for local injection; most commonly the 25 gauge (0.5 mm) is used. Larger needles, such as 21 or 19 gauge, may be used for aspiration. The optimal length generally is 1.5 inches, which allows adequate penetration for most soft tissue injections. Spinal needles, which are 3 inches in length (22 or 23 gauge), occasionally are useful for trochanteric bursal injections in obese individuals. Tuberculin syringes are especially useful for injection of small structures, such as flexor tendon sheaths.

Injection Techniques

SUBACROMIAL BURSAL INJECTION

Equipment

A 1-mL syringe, 25-gauge 1.5-inch needle, 40 to 60 mg methyl-prednisolone.

Approach

Palpate the tip of the acromion and the greater tuberosity of the humerus with the patient sitting. The subacromial space lies between these two structures. The needle should be advanced just under the tip of the acromion in a slightly upward direction and in the direction of the scapular spine (Fig. 10.1).

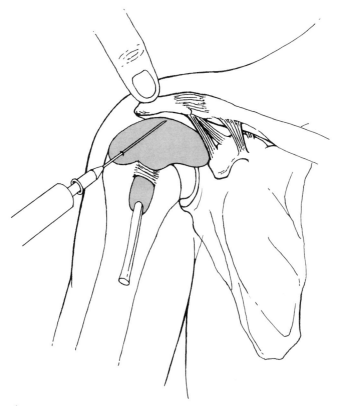

Figure 10.1 Subacromial bursal injection.

Injection Techniques

BICEPS TENDON INJECTION

Equipment

A 1-mL syringe, 25-gauge 1.5-inch needle, 40 to 60 mg methylprednisolone.

Approach

Palpate the long head of the biceps tendon within the bicipital groove. Insert the needle into the tendon and then pull back to a point where there is no significant resistance to compression of the plunger of the syringe. This will deposit corticosteroid around the vicinity of the tendon sheath. Too much resistance may indicate that the needle is still in the tendon itself, and forced compression of the plunger runs the risk of deposition in the tendon itself, which can produce rupture (Fig. 10.2).

ASPIRATION OF THE OLECRANON BURSA

Equipment

A 5-mL syringe, 19-gauge 1.5-inch needle.

Approach

Palpate the tip of the elbow to isolate the olecranon bursa. Insert the needle into the bursa into its medial or lateral side. Aspiration of the bursa at its apex may leave a draining sinus tract (Fig. 10.3).

LATERAL EPICONDYLITIS INJECTION

Equipment

A 1-mL syringe, 25-gauge 1.5-inch needle, 20 to 40 mg methylprednisolone.

Approach

With the elbow flexed, identify the point of maximal tenderness (usually just distal and slightly superior to the lateral epicondyle). Insert the needle at 90 degrees to the skin surface. Inject the contents of the syringe with approximately $\frac{1}{2}$ to 1 inch of the needle into the tissue (Fig. 10.4).

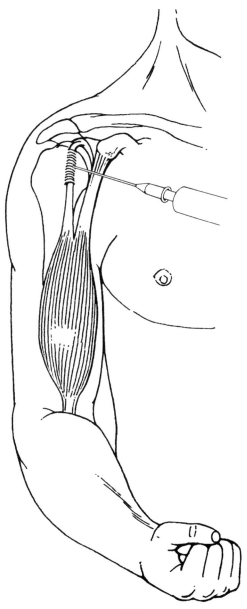

Figure 10.2 Injection for bicipital tendonitis.

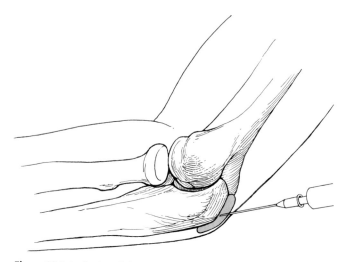

Figure 10.3 Aspiration of the olecranon bursa.

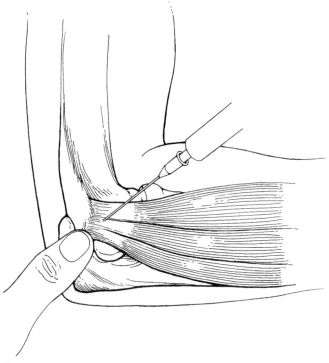

Figure 10.4 Lateral epicondylitis injection.

Injection Techniques

CARPAL TUNNEL INJECTION

Equipment

A 1-mL syringe, 25-gauge 1.5-inch needle, 20 to 40 mg methyl-prednisolone.

Approach

Isolate the flexor carpi ulnaris tendon with resistive flexion of the wrist. Insert the needle just to the ulnar side of the flexor carpi ulnaris tendon at an angle of 60 degrees with the needle pointed toward the fingers (Fig. 10.5).

FINGER FLEXOR TENDON INJECTION

Equipment

A 1-mL syringe, 25-gauge 1.5-inch needle, 10 to 20 mg methyl-prednisolone.

Approach

Palpate the nodule on the flexor tendon of the symptomatic, triggering finger. Typically the nodule lies over the metacarpophalangeal joint. Insert the needle into the nodule, then ask the patient to gently flex the finger. If the syringe moves (indicating that the needle is within the tendon), withdraw the needle until there is no movement of the syringe with finger flexion and then compress the plunger of the syringe (Fig. 10.6).

DE QUERVAIN'S TENOSYNOVITIS INJECTION

Equipment

A 1-mL syringe, 25-gauge 1.5-inch needle, 10 to 20 mg methyl-prednisolone.

Approach

Isolate the common extensor tendon complex (combined sheath of the abductor pollicis longus and extensor pollicis brevis tendons) of the thumb. Insert the needle at approximately 45 degrees, pointed toward the antecubital fossa. Ask the patient to gently extend the thumb. If the syringe moves (indicating that the needle is within the tendon), withdraw the needle until there is no movement of the sy-

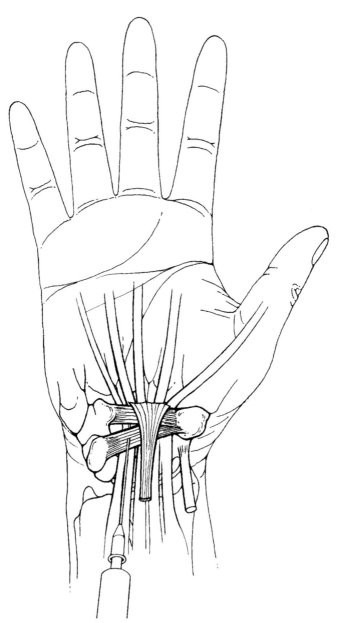

Figure 10.5 Carpal tunnel injection.

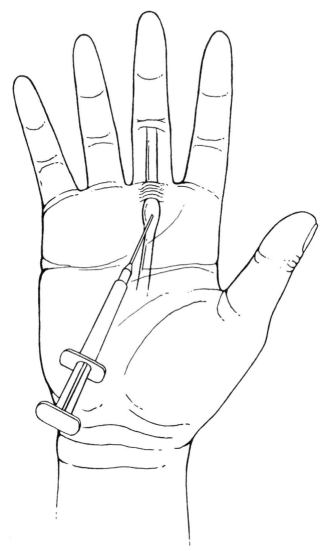

Figure 10.6 Finger flexor tendon injection.

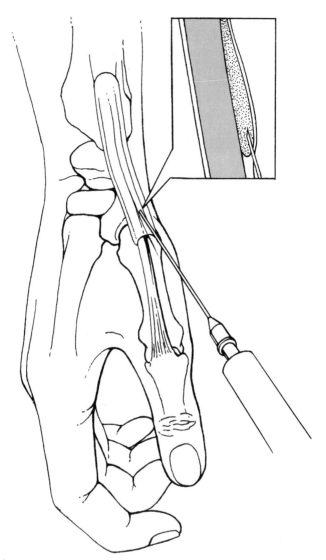

Figure 10.7 de Quervain's tenosynovitis injection.

ringe with thumb extension and then compress the plunger of the syringe (Fig. 10.7).

TROCHANTERIC BURSAL INJECTION

Equipment

A 1-mL or 3-mL syringe, 25-gauge 1.5-inch needle or 22-gauge 3.0-inch spinal needle, 40 to 80 mg methylprednisolone.

Approach

Position the patient on the asymptomatic side. Identify the greater trochanter and the point of maximum tenderness (usually just posterior to the most lateral extent of the greater trochanter). Insert the needle at 90 degrees to the skin and advance to the periosteum of the greater trochanter. Withdraw the needle slightly and inject (Fig. 10.8).

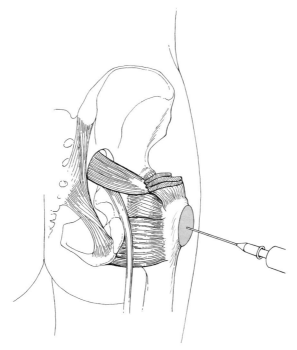

Figure 10.8 Trochanteric bursal injection.

Injection Techniques

ANSERINE BURSAL INJECTION

Equipment

A 1-mL syringe, 25-gauge 1.5-inch needle, 20 to 40 mg methyl-prednisolone.

Approach

With the patient supine, identify the anserine bursa just distal to the medial joint line of the knee. Insert the needle at 90 degrees to the skin and advance to the periosteum of the tibia. Withdraw the needle slightly and then inject (Fig. 10.9).

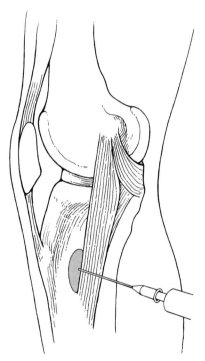

Figure 10.9 Anserine bursal injection.

Subject Index

101

Subject Index

Subject Index

Subject Index